English Public Speaking for Medical Purpose

医学英语演讲赏析

主 编 王 蕾 薄蓉蓉

编 者（按姓名首字母排序）

顾亚琳 陆丽英

秦 晔 项菊仟

张之薇

南京大学出版社

图书在版编目(CIP)数据

医学英语演讲赏析 / 王蕾,薄蓉蓉主编. — 南京：
南京大学出版社,2019.6(2021.7 重印)
ISBN 978 - 7 - 305 - 21803 - 3

Ⅰ. ①医… Ⅱ. ①王… ②薄… Ⅲ. ①医学－英语－
演讲 Ⅳ. ①R

中国版本图书馆 CIP 数据核字(2019)第 051072 号

出版发行 南京大学出版社
社　　址 南京市汉口路 22 号　　　　邮　编　210093
出 版 人 金鑫荣
书　　名 **医学英语演讲赏析**
主　　编 王　蕾　薄蓉蓉
责任编辑 裴维维　　　　　　编辑热线　025 - 83592123
照　　排 南京南琳图文制作有限公司
印　　刷 南京人民印刷厂有限责任公司
开　　本 787×960　1/16　印张 12.5　字数 310 千
版　　次 2019 年 6 月第 1 版　2021 年 7 月第 2 次印刷
ISBN 978 - 7 - 305 - 21803 - 3
定　　价 37.00 元

网址：http://www.njupco.com
官方微博：http://weibo.com/njupco
微信服务号：njuyuexue
销售咨询热线：(025) 83594756

前　言

在"一带一路"的背景下，人才强国战略深入实施。时代和社会发展需要进一步提高国民的综合素质，培养具有国际视野的创新人才。这些变化和需求对课程改革和人才培养提出了新的要求，要求高校能提供培养学生国际交流能力的课程，使他们能承担起国家对外交流的任务，而英语演讲课程就是有效培养学生这一能力的课程之一。研究表明，英语演讲课程可以全面提高学生综合运用英语语言的能力，提高学生的文化修养、批判性思维能力和审美能力。

近年来，伴随着医学教育的国际化进程，国家对涉外医学人才的需求越来越大，这对医学院校的英语课程设置提出了更高的要求。医学院校的英语课程不仅要帮助医学生打好语言基础，更要注重培养医学生实际应用语言的能力，尤其是用英语在专业领域开展有效交际的能力。因此，在医学院校开设英语演讲课程，符合医学院校英语教学改革的需求，有利于卓越医学人才的培养。

医学院校的英语演讲课程在设计理据、教学模块等方面可遵循通识类演讲课程设置的一般规律，但在教学内容和教学资源的选择上，则应凸显医学院校自身的人才培养目标和学校特色。在这样的背景下，本教程应运而生。

本教程考虑到了医学院校英语教学中医学性与人文性的统一。选取的演讲材料既包括针对疫苗、基因等医学专业问题的论述，又包括针对触诊、临终关怀等医学人文话题的讨论，体现了医学英语材料的可靠性与时效性。本教程选取的演讲以近年来 TED 演讲资源为主，演讲者从专业的角度呈现了医学研究领域的最新进展及其对医学发展的探索和思考。教程中选取的演讲涵盖了说解性演讲(informative speech)、说服性演讲(persuasive speech)等常见的英语演讲形式,并深度评析了演讲者在演讲过程中所使用的策略。学习者可以根据自身的专业特点和实际水平,有选择性地将这些演讲技巧运用在具有个人风格的英语公共演讲当中。

本教程由14个单元组成,每个单元包含 Speech 1、Speech 2 两个演讲,其中 Speech 1 为精讲材料,Speech 2 为拓展材料。每个演讲的标题下方附有一个二维码,学习者可以扫描二维码,观看演讲视频。

Speech 1 版块主要由以下三个部分构成:

1. 演讲者简介

这个部分概述了演讲者的背景资料,重点介绍了演讲者的学习经历和职业背景,体现了演讲者的信誉度(credibility)。

2. 英文演讲稿及其中文译文

这个部分呈现了演讲稿原文及其中文译文,便于学习者对讲稿的结构、措辞展开细致地分析。为了使学习者更好地理解和掌握演讲的关键信息,编者将该演讲中出现的医学英语高频词汇集中在生词表罗列。

3. 演讲赏析

这个部分在演讲类型、讲稿结构、语言的生动与适切、视觉辅助手段、演讲风格与策略等方面对该演讲展开了详尽地分析,理论的观点参考了 Stephen E. Lucas《演讲的艺术》(第十版)一书。

Speech 2 版块名为"精彩加油站",作为 Speech 1 版块的补充和拓展。

本教程选取的演讲涉及医生的关怀、埃博拉病毒、大脑的自我修复、基因革命、寄生虫的逆袭等话题,科普性与趣味性兼具,难度适中,适合已经开展了医学专业课程学习的医学院校中、高年级学生使用,也适合具有涉外学术演说需求的医务工作者使用。

南京大学陈萱老师对本书提出了许多修改意见,在此表示感谢。

编 者

2019 年 6 月

目　录

Lecture 1　A Doctor's Touch 医生的关怀 ···································· 1

精彩加油站：Got a Meeting? Take a Walk 要开会？边走边谈 ········· 18

Lecture 2　What You Need to Know About Ebola 你们需要了解的关于埃博拉的事情 ·· 21

精彩加油站：Why Genetic Research Must Be More Diverse 人类基因研究需要更多样化 ··· 27

Lecture 3　The Brain May Be Able to Repair Itself—With Help 大脑也许可以在辅助下进行自我修复 ··· 32

精彩加油站：This Gel Can Make You Stop Bleeding Instantly 可以立即止血的凝胶 ··· 41

Lecture 4　Welcome to the Genomic Revolution 欢迎进入基因革命时代 ········ 45

精彩加油站：Your Genes Are Not Your Fate 基因决定不了你的命运 ··· 57

Lecture 5　Zombie Roaches and Other Parasite Tales 寄生虫的逆袭 ············· 61

精彩加油站：Could We Cure HIV with Lasers? 我们能用激光治疗艾滋病吗？ ··· 73

Lecture 6　The Next Outbreak? We're Not Ready 下一次疫情暴发,我们准备好了吗？ ··· 76

精彩加油站：Plague Doctor in the 17th Century 17 世纪的瘟疫医生 ··· 85

Lecture 7　Alzheimer's Is Not Normal Aging—and We Can Cure It 阿尔茨海默病不是正常衰老的必然结果——我们可以治愈它 ······················· 88

精彩加油站：Weekly Address: Celebrating Fifty Years of Medicare and

Medicaid 美国总统奥巴马每周演讲：庆祝医疗保险和医疗补助制度实施 50 周年 ·· 96

Lecture 8   A Second Opinion on Developmental Disorders 关于学习障碍的新认识 ·· 100

精彩加油站：The Best Gift I Ever Survived 我收到最好的礼物 ······ 107

Lecture 9   What's So Funny About Mental Illness? 精神病有什么可笑的？ ······ 110

精彩加油站：Programming Bacteria to Detect Cancer（and Maybe Treat it）利用细菌发现癌症（也许还能治愈它）································ 119

Lecture 10   The Mystery of Chronic Pain 慢性疼痛之谜 ····················· 123

精彩加油站：Peng Liyuan's Speech in Geneva 彭丽媛在瑞士日内瓦出席 亲善大使任期续延暨颁奖仪式上的致辞 ·································· 132

Lecture 11   The Spellbinding Art of Human Anatomy 人体解剖——引人入胜的艺 术 ··· 136

精彩加油站：On the Virtual Dissection Table 谈谈虚拟解剖台 ······ 147

Lecture 12   The Troubling Reason Why Vaccines Are Made Too Late 为什么疫苗姗 姗来迟？ ··· 150

精彩加油站：Weekly Address：Taking Action Against the Zika Virus 美 国总统奥巴马每周演讲——采取行动抗击塞卡病毒 ················ 157

Lecture 13   Why Medicine Often Has Dangerous Side Effects for Women 药物对女 性的副作用 ·· 162

精彩加油站：Weekly Address：Trump's Attack on Obamacare 美国总统 特朗普每周演讲：废除奥巴马医改方案 ······························· 174

Lecture 14   What Makes Life Worth Living in the Face of Death 当死亡降临 ·· 177

精彩加油站："Am I dying?" The Honest Answer "我快死了吗？"一个诚 实的回答 ··· 190

Lecture 1　A Doctor's Touch
医生的关怀

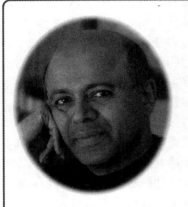

　　亚伯拉罕·维基斯(Abraham Verghese)是一位印度裔的美国内科医生,同时也是一位畅销书作家。从医学院毕业前,他曾在医院做过一年的清洁工。正是这段经历,让他从人的角度来重新认识病人,也促成他开始写作。他在德克萨斯圣安东尼奥大学成立了医学人文伦理中心,中心的宗旨就是"想象病人的经历"。2011年,他当选为美国医学研究所(Institute of Medicine)成员。2015年,他被奥巴马授予美国国家人文奖章。现在,他是斯坦福医学院医学理论与实践方向的教授、内科医学系高级副主任。

1　A few months ago, a 40 year-old woman came to an emergency room in a hospital close to where I live, and she was brought in confused. Her blood pressure was an alarming 230 over 170. Within a few minutes, she went into *cardiac collapse*①. She was *resuscitated*②, stabilized, *whisked*③ over to a CAT scan suite right next to the emergency room, because they were concerned about *blood clots*④ in the lung. And the CAT scan revealed no blood clots in the lung, but it showed *bilateral*⑤, visible, *palpable*⑥ breast masses, breast tumors, that had *metastasized*⑦ widely all over the body. And the real tragedy was, if you look through her records, she had been seen in four or five other health care institutions in the preceding two years. Four or five opportunities to see the breast masses, touch the breast mass, intervene at a much earlier stage than when we saw her.

2　Ladies and gentlemen, that is not an unusual story. Unfortunately, it happens all the time. I joke, but I only half joke, that if you come to one of our hospitals missing a limb, no one will

1　几个月前,一位 40 岁的女士来到医院急诊室。这个医院离我住的地方不远。她来的时候神志不清,血压处于警戒值:收缩压 230,舒张压 170。几分钟内她就昏迷了。被救醒后,她的情况开始稳定下来。因为医生担心她的肺部有血块,她被带到急诊室旁边的扫描室进行 CAT 扫描。结果显示她的肺部并没有血块,但是胸部两侧有清晰可见的肿块,是乳腺肿瘤,并且已经转移到全身各部位。真正悲剧的是,如果你查看她的记录会发现,在过去的两年里,她已经辗转去过四五家医疗机构了。这就意味着这些乳腺肿瘤本来有四五次的机会可以通过触检发现,而医生本可以在更早些时候介入治疗。

2　诸位,这不是特例。很不幸,这样的事一直在发生。我常会和人开玩笑地说——或者都不能完全算是玩笑——假如你缺胳膊少

① cardiac collapse 心脏崩溃
② resuscitate *v.* 使复苏,复兴
③ whisk *v.* 搅拌,挥动
④ blood clot 血块
⑤ bilateral *adj.* 双边的,两侧的
⑥ palpable *adj.* 可感知的,明显的
⑦ metastasize *v.* 转移

believe you till they get a CAT scan, MRI or *orthopedic*① consult. I am not a Luddite. I teach at Stanford. I'm a physician practicing with cutting-edge technology. But I'd like to make the case to you in the next 17 minutes that when we shortcut the physical exam, when we lean towards ordering tests instead of talking to and examining the patient, we not only overlook simple diagnoses that can be diagnosed at a treatable, early stage, but we're losing much more than that. We're losing a ritual. We're losing a ritual that I believe is transformative, transcendent, and is at the heart of the patient-physician relationship. This may actually be *heresy*② to say this at TED, but I'd like to introduce you to the most important innovation, I think, in medicine to come in the next 10 years, and that is the power of the human hand—to touch, to comfort, to diagnose and to bring about treatment.

3 I'd like to introduce you first to this person whose image you may or may not recognize. This is Sir Arthur Conan Doyle. Since we're in Edinburgh, I'm a big fan of Conan Doyle. You might not know that Conan Doyle went to medical school here in Edinburgh, and his character, Sherlock Holmes, was inspired by

腿去了医院，除非你做了 CAT 扫描、磁共振成像和骨科诊断，否则没人会相信你缺胳膊少腿的事实。我并不是反对技术进步的勒德分子，我在斯坦福大学教书，同时还是个掌握尖端技术的内科医生。但在接下来的 17 分钟里，我想告诉你们的是，当我们缩减检查环节，给病人开上一堆化验单，而不再通过问诊和触诊了解病情时，我们错失的就不仅仅是易于诊断和治疗疾病早期了。我们错过的是一套医疗的仪式，是一套我认为可以摧枯拉朽、超越一切的医疗仪式，而这正是医患关系的核心所在。在 TED 讲这个内容可能有点不合时宜，但我想向各位介绍的是，在未来的十年里，医学最重要的变革就是关注人类之手的力量——关爱、抚慰、诊断和治疗的力量。

3 首先我想介绍一个人，你们不一定认得出他。这是亚瑟·柯南·道尔爵士。我们现在身处爱丁堡，那你们也许有人会知道柯南·道尔是在爱丁堡上的医学院吧。我本人是柯南·道尔的超级粉丝。而他正是在这儿受到一位

---

① orthopedic *adj.* 整形手术的
② heresy *n.* 异端

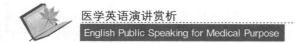

Sir Joseph Bell. Joseph Bell was an extraordinary teacher by all accounts. And Conan Doyle, writing about Bell, described the following exchange between Bell and his students.

4   So picture Bell sitting in the outpatient department, students all around him, patients signing up in the emergency room and being registered and being brought in. And a woman comes in with a child, and Conan Doyle describes the following exchange. The woman says, "Good Morning." Bell says, "What sort of crossing did you have on the *ferry*① from Burntisland?" She says, "It was good." And he says, "What did you do with the other child?" She says, "I left him with my sister at Leith." And he says, "And did you take the shortcut down Inverleith Row to get here to the *infirmary*②?" She says, "I did." And he says, "Would you still be working at the linoleum factory?" And she says, "I am."

5   And Bell then goes on to explain to the students. He says, "You see, when she said, 'Good morning,' I picked up her Fife accent. And the nearest ferry crossing from Fife is from Burntisland. And so she must have taken

异常杰出的老师约瑟夫·贝尔的启发，创作了笔下的著名人物——福尔摩斯。柯南·道尔曾对这位老师和他的学生之间的交流做过如下的描述。

4   贝尔坐在门诊部里，他的学生围绕在他身旁。病人们在急诊室里进行登记、挂号，然后被依次带进来。一个带小孩的女士走了进来。柯南·道尔这样记叙他们之间的交谈："女人说：'早上好。'贝尔问：'你从本泰兰坐渡船过来一路还好吗？'她说：'挺好的。'贝尔又问：'你的另一个孩子呢？'她答：'我拜托住在利斯的姐姐照顾了。'贝尔接着问：'那你来诊所走了印佛里斯那条近路了吧？'她回答：'没错。'贝尔再问道：'你还打算在油毡厂继续干活吗？'她说：'是的。'"

5   然后贝尔向他的学生解释说："当她说'你好'的时候，我听出她的法伊夫口音。而离法伊夫最近的渡船是在本泰兰，所以我推测出她是从那里过来的。你们

① ferry *n.* 渡船
② infirmary *n.* 医务室，医院

the ferry over. You notice that the coat she's carrying is too small for the child who is with her, and therefore, she started out the journey with two children, but dropped one off along the way. You notice the clay on the *soles*① of her feet. Such red clay is not found within a hundred miles of Edinburgh, except in the *botanical gardens*②. And therefore, she took a short cut down Inverleith Row to arrive here. And finally, she has a *dermatitis*③ on the fingers of her right hand, a dermatitis that is unique to the linoleum factory workers in Burntisland." And when Bell actually *strips*④ the patient, begins to examine the patient, you can only imagine how much more he would *discern*⑤. And as a teacher of medicine, as a student myself, I was so inspired by that story.

6　But you might not realize that our ability to look into the body in this simple way, using our senses, is quite recent. The picture I'm showing you is of Leopold Auenbrugger who, in the late 1700s, discovered *percussion*⑥. And the story is that Leopold Auenbrugger was the son of an innkeeper. And his father used to go down into the basement to tap on the sides of casks of

也注意到她拿着的外套了吧。这件外套对她身旁的小孩来说太小了。所以她肯定带了两个孩子，路上放下了一个。还有她鞋底上的泥，爱丁堡方圆百里内没有这种红泥，除了植物园。所以她肯定是从印佛里斯抄近路来这儿的。最后，她右手手指有皮炎，这种皮炎只有本泰兰油毡厂的工人会得。"然后贝尔就让她脱了衣服开始检查。他对事物的观察判断能力几乎让人难以置信。作为一名医学老师，同时也是一个学生，这个故事让我深受启发。

6　也许你们还不知道，我们利用感官给病人检查身体虽然看上去操作简单，却是近代的发明。这张照片上的人是利奥波德·奥恩布鲁格，他在 18 世纪末发明了叩诊法。据说利奥波德·奥恩布鲁格的父亲是个旅馆老板，他常去地下室的酒窖，通过敲击酒桶

---

①　sole *n.* 脚底
②　botanical gardens 植物园
③　dermatitis *n.* 皮炎
④　strip *v.* 剥光
⑤　discern *v.* 了解，识别
⑥　percussion *n.* 敲打，碰撞

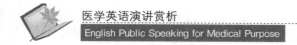

wine to determine how much wine was left and whether to reorder. And so when Auenbrugger became a physician, he began to do the same thing. He began to tap on the chests of his patients, on their *abdomens*①. And basically everything we know about percussion, which you can think of as an *ultrasound*② of its day—organ enlargement, fluid around the heart, fluid in the lungs, abdominal changes—all of this he described in this wonderful manuscript "Inventum Novum," "New Invention," which would have disappeared into obscurity, except for the fact that this physician, Corvisart, a famous French physician—famous only because he was a physician to this gentleman (a picture of Napoleon is shown on the screen)—Corvisart repopularized and reintroduced the work.

来判断桶里还剩多少酒，要不要追加订单。所以当奥恩布鲁格成了内科医生的时候，他也开始使用这种方法。他叩击病人的胸腔，还有腹部。在他的伟大的著作《新发明》里，他记录了基本上我们所了解的一切叩诊的应用，包括确诊器官增大、心肺积水、腹部变化等，这在当时几乎等同于现在的超声波技术。这份手稿几近失传，多亏了一位叫作科维扎卡的法国医生，奥恩布鲁格的这部著作才得以重见天日并逐渐普及。可当时这位医生出名却只是因为他在给这位先生当医生（幻灯片上显示拿破仑的照片。）

7　And it was followed a year or two later by Laennec discovering the *stethoscope*③. Laennec, it is said, was walking in the streets of Paris and saw two children playing with a stick. One was scratching at the end of the stick, another child listened at the other end. And Laennec thought this would be a wonderful way to listen to the chest or listen to the abdomen using what he called "the cylinder." Later he renamed it the stethoscope. And that

7　一两年后，莱尼克发明了听诊器。据说莱尼克走在巴黎的街上时，看见两个小孩在玩一根棍子，其中一个孩子挠棍子的一头，让另一个孩子在棍子的那头听声音。莱尼克认为用这个他称之为"圆筒"的仪器听胸腔和腹腔是个很不错的主意。后来他把这个"圆筒"命名为听诊器。这就是听诊器和听诊法的由来。于是在

①　abdomen *n.* 腹部，腹腔
②　ultrasound *n.* 超声波
③　stethoscope *n.* 听诊器

is how stethoscope and *auscultation*① was born. So within a few years, in the late 1800s, early 1900s, all of a sudden, the barber surgeon had given way to the physician who was trying to make a diagnosis. If you'll recall, prior to that time, no matter what *ailed*② you, you went to see the barber surgeon who wound up cupping you, bleeding you, purging you. And, oh yes, if you wanted, he would give you a haircut—short on the sides, long in the back—and pull your tooth while he was at it. He made no attempt at diagnosis. In fact, some of you might well know that the barber pole, the red and white stripes, represents the blood bandages of the barber surgeon, and the *receptacles*③ on either end represent the pots in which the blood was collected. But the arrival of auscultation and percussion represented a sea change, a moment when physicians were beginning to look inside the body.

8   And this particular painting, I think, represents the pinnacle, the peak, of that clinical era. This is a very famous painting: "The Doctor" by Luke Fildes. Luke Fildes was commissioned to paint this by Tate, who then established the Tate Gallery. And Tate asked Fildes to paint a painting of social importance.

19 世纪末 20 世纪初的几年时间内,能够给病人诊断的内科医生一夜之间取代了外科理发师(从前能实行外科治疗的理发师)。你可能还记得,在那之前,不管你病得多厉害,到了外科理发师那儿,他们只会给你拔罐,给你放血,给你冲洗。当然如果你愿意的话,他们也给你理个发,两边短后边长,还顺便给你拔个牙,完全没有诊断的环节。也许有些人还记得理发店红白两色旋转的招牌,那红白条纹象征止血的绷带,两侧的容器则代表收集血液的壶。听诊法和叩诊法的出现代表着一个巨大的变化,意味着内科医生开始探视人体的内部。

8   我认为这幅画代表着那个时代医疗水平的顶峰。这是幅非常著名的油画,卢克·菲尔德斯的《医生》。这是一幅受泰特之托创作的作品。泰特当时成立了泰特美术馆,于是他请卢克·菲尔德斯创作一幅能体现社会意义的

---

① auscultation *n.* 听诊
② ail *v.* 生病,感到不舒服
③ receptacle *n.* 容器

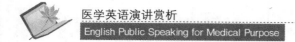
And it's interesting that Fildes picked this topic. Fildes' oldest son, Philip, died at the age of nine on Christmas Eve after a brief illness. And Fildes was so taken by the physician who held *vigil*① at the bedside for two, three nights, that he decided that he would try and depict the physician in our time—almost a *tribute*② to this physician. And hence the painting "The Doctor," a very famous painting. It's been on calendars, postage stamps in many different countries. I've often wondered, what would Fildes have done had he been asked to paint this painting in the modern era, in the year 2011? Would he have substituted a computer screen for where he had the patient?

9　I've gotten into some trouble in Silicon Valley for saying that the patient in the bed has almost become an icon for the real patient who's in the computer. I've actually coined a term for that entity in the computer. I call it the iPatient. The iPatient is getting wonderful care all across America. The real patient often wonders, where is everyone? When are they going to come by and explain things to me? Who's in charge? There's a real *disjunction*③ between the patient's perception and our own

画,有趣的是菲尔德斯选择了医生这个主题。菲利普是菲尔德斯的大儿子,他9岁的时候生了一场小病却最终不治死于平安夜。菲尔德斯被那位在病床旁守了两三夜的医生深深感动,于是他决定试着描绘出那个时代的医生——用以表示对那位医生的敬意。《医生》这幅名画出现在很多国家的挂历和邮票上。我常想,如果菲尔德斯在2011年被要求画这幅画,他会怎么办? 画里的患者是不是得换成电脑显示器了?

9　躺在病床上的病人形象几乎只成为通过计算机问诊病人的符号,因为这个说法我还在硅谷惹出了些麻烦。事实上我为那些在电脑里问诊的病人取了一个新名字"电子病人"。全美国的"电子病人"都得到很好的治疗。可现实中的病人却常常感到困惑:人都去哪儿了? 他们什么时候来给我解释这些玩意儿? 有没有人负责啊? 对于什么是最佳医疗这个

---

① vigil *n.* 守夜,熬夜
② tribute *n.* 致敬,贡品
③ disjunction *n.* 分离

perceptions as physicians of the best medical care.

问题,病人和医生的想法存在着巨大的差异。

10　I want to show you a picture of what rounds looked like when I was in training. The focus was around the patient. We went from bed to bed. The attending physician was in charge. Too often these days rounds look very much like this, where the discussion is taking place in a room far away from the patient. The discussion is all about images on the computer, data. And the one critical piece missing is that of the patient.

10　我想向你们展示一下,我当年的临床实习是什么样的。在主治医师的带领下,我们从一张病床到另一张病床,我们的工作重心是围绕病人展开的。可现如今的临床实习却往往是这样的:大家在一个远离病人的房间里,围绕电脑上的图像和数据展开讨论。整个过程里最重要的部分已经缺失,那就是病人。

11　Now I've been influenced in this thinking by two anecdotes that I want to share with you. One had to do with a friend of mine who had a breast cancer, had a small breast cancer detected—had her *lumpectomy*① in the town in which I lived. This is when I was in Texas. And she then spent a lot of time researching to find the best cancer center in the world to get her subsequent care. And she found the place and decided to go there, went there. Which is why I was surprised a few months later to see her back in our own town, getting her subsequent care with her private *oncologist*②.

11　还有两件对我触动很大的事,我想与你们分享一下。我有一个患有乳腺癌的朋友,在发现一个小的乳腺肿瘤后,她在我住的那个城市做了肿瘤切除手术。那时我在德克萨斯。然后她花了很长时间寻找世界上最好的癌症中心,接受后续治疗。她找到了,然后去了。几个月后,我很惊讶地看见她回来了,在她的私人医生那里进行术后康复。

---

① lumpectomy *n.* 乳房肿块切除术
② oncologist *n.* 肿瘤学家

12   And I pressed her, and I asked her, "Why did you come back and get your care here?" And she was reluctant to tell me. She said, "The cancer center was wonderful. It had a beautiful facility, giant atrium, valet parking, a piano that played itself, a concierge that took you around from here to there. But," she said, "but, they did not touch my breasts." Now you and I could argue that they probably did not need to touch her breasts. They had her scanned inside out. They understood her breast cancer at the molecular level; they had no need to touch her breasts.

13   But to her, it mattered deeply. It was enough for her to make the decision to get her subsequent care with her private oncologist who, every time she went, examined both breasts including the *axillary*① tail, examined her axilla carefully, examined her *cervical*② region, her *inguinal*③ region, did a thorough exam. And to her, that spoke of a kind of attentiveness that she needed. I was very influenced by that anecdote.

14   I was also influenced by another experience that I had, again, when I was in Texas, before

12   我问她："你为什么回来接受康复治疗?"她好像不太愿意细讲,只是说:"那个癌症中心非常棒,设施一流。大堂很宽敞,有服务生停车,有自动弹奏的钢琴,有人带你到处溜达。但是他们根本没碰我的胸部。"当然我们现在可以进行争辩,他们也许没有必要碰她的胸部,扫描就可以搞得一清二楚了。他们可以从分子层面了解她的乳腺癌,所以没有必要触诊。

13   但对她来说,这很重要。这足够让她做出回到私人医生那里接受康复治疗的决定。每次去,她的私人医生都会检查她的两侧乳房直至腋尾,还会仔细检查腋窝、颈部和腹股沟。对她来说,这样全面的检查正是她所需要的关注。这件事深深影响了我。

14   另外一段经历同样给我印象深刻。那也是我在德克萨斯时的

① axillary *n.* 腋窝
② cervical *adj.* 颈部的
③ inguinal *adj.* 腹股沟的

I moved to Stanford. I had a reputation as being interested in patients with chronic fatigue. This is not a reputation you would wish on your worst enemy. I say that because these are difficult patients. They have often been rejected by their families, have had bad experiences with medical care and they come to you fully prepared for you to join the long list of people who's about to disappoint them. And I learned very early on with my first patient that I could not do justice to this very complicated patient with all the records they were bringing in and a new patient visit of 45 minutes. There was just no way. And if I tried, I'd disappoint them.

15　　And so I hit on this method where I invited the patient to tell me the story for their entire first visit，and I tried not to interrupt them. We know the average American physician interrupts their patient in 14 seconds. And if I ever get to heaven，it will be because I held my piece for 45 minutes and did not interrupt my patient. I then scheduled the physical exam for two weeks hence，and when the patient came for the physical，I was able to do a thorough physical，because I had nothing else to do. I like to think that I do a thorough physical exam，but because the whole visit was now about the physical，I could do an extraordinarily thorough exam.

事儿，那会儿我还没搬到斯坦福。大家都知道我非常关注有慢性疲劳症状的病人，但这绝对不是什么好事儿。我这么说是因为这些病人都比较难缠。他们经常被家人排斥，有很多不顺心的就诊经历。他们到你这儿之前就想好，你可能会是下一个令他们失望的人。我从看见我的第一个病人起，就已经意识到，想在45分钟的初诊时间内，对这些有着复杂治疗记录的病人做出合理诊断是很困难的。这绝对做不到。如果我做出了诊断，那我就会成为下一个令他们失望的人。

15　所以我想到了一个办法，那就是在他们初诊的整个阶段，完全听他们的自述，尽量不打断他们。大家都知道，美国医生平均每14秒就会打断一次病人的叙述。我想将来如果我能进天堂的话，那肯定是因为我做到了四十五分钟不间断的聆听。然后我会在两周后安排一次体检。那时候，我唯一能做的事也就是对病人进行一次彻底的身体检查了。因为这次就医就是为体检而来的，所以叫彻底检查都不够，应该称之为细致入微的仔细检查吧。

16　　And I remember my very first patient in that series continued to tell me more history during what was meant to be the physical exam visit. And I began my ritual. I always begin with the pulse, then I examine the hands, then I look at the nail beds, then I slide my hand up to the *epitrochlear node*①, and I was into my ritual. And when my ritual began, this very voluble patient began to quiet down. And I remember having a very *eerie*② sense that the patient and I had slipped back into a primitive ritual in which I had a role and the patient had a role. And when I was done, the patient said to me with some awe, "I have never been examined like this before." Now if that were true, it's a true condemnation of our health care system, because they had been seen in other places.

17　　I then proceeded to tell the patient, once the patient was dressed, the standard things that the person must have heard in other institutions, which is, "This is not in your head. This is real. The good news, it's not

16　我记得我的第一个慢性疲劳症病人在这个过程中,又陆陆续续给我讲述了很多病史,尽管这次就诊本来是以身体检查为主的。我开始了我的例行检查动作。我总是从测脉搏开始,然后检查手,接下来看甲床,随后把手慢慢移至肱骨内上髁淋巴结的位置,我的例行操作一步步地进行着。随着触诊的展开,这位健谈的病人也慢慢安静下来。我记得自己产生了一种很奇怪的感觉,我们似乎又回到了过去,重温了一套最原始的治疗仪式,在这套仪式中医生和病人都找到了各自的角色。当我完成检查的时候,病人对我敬畏地说:"我从来没被这样检查过。"如果真是这样,那无疑是对我们的医疗体系最真实的谴责,因为他去过很多医院,却从未享受过如此待遇。

17　等病人穿戴完毕,我接着告诉他一些其他医疗机构也会告诉他的内容:"这不是你想象出来的,这是真的。好消息是,你得的不是癌症,不是肺结核,不是球孢子菌病或者什么真菌感染。坏消

---

① epitrochlear node 肱骨内上髁淋巴结
② eerie *adj.* 怪异的

cancer, it's not *tuberculosis*①, it's not *coccidioidomycosis*② or some obscure *fungal*③ infection. The bad news is we don't know exactly what's causing this, but here's what you should do, here's what we should do." And I would lay out all the standard treatment options that the patient had heard elsewhere.

息是我们不清楚这是什么导致的。这些……是你可以做的，这些……是我们可以做的。"接着我会给病人列出若干治疗选项，其实这些都是他在其他地方也曾听到过的标准化建议。

18　And I always felt that if my patient gave up the quest for the magic doctor, the magic treatment and began with me on a course towards wellness, it was because I had earned the right to tell them these things by virtue of the examination. Something of importance had *transpired*④ in the exchange. I took this to my colleagues at Stanford in anthropology and told them the same story. And they immediately said to me, "Well, you are describing a classic ritual." And they helped me understand that rituals are all about transformation.

18　我总觉得，如果我的病人放弃寻求神医或神奇疗法的尝试，而转投我寻求健康，那一定是因为这种一丝不苟的检查，为我的医嘱赢得了更多的说服力。某种关键性的变化在我们交流的过程中已经不知不觉地发生了。我把同样的故事告诉了斯坦福大学研究人类学的同事们。他们立刻对我说："你说的正是一个典型的仪式。"他们接着给我解释了仪式和转变的关系。

19　We marry, for example, with great pomp and ceremony and expense to signal our departure from a life of solitude and misery and loneliness to one of eternal bliss. I'm not sure why you're laughing. That was the original

19　举例说，我们结婚时，会用舞会、仪式和昂贵的花销来告别孤独、寂寞的悲惨生活，迎接永恒的幸福。我不知道你们为什么笑。我们结婚原本是这么希望的，对

---

①　tuberculosis *n.* 肺结核
②　coccidioidomycosis *n.* 球孢子菌病
③　fungal *adj.* 真菌的
④　transpire *v.* 使蒸发，排出

intent, was it not? We signal transitions of power with rituals. We signal the passage of a life with rituals. Rituals are terribly important. They're all about transformation. Well, I would submit to you that the ritual of one individual coming to another and telling them things that they would not tell their preacher or rabbi, and then, incredibly on top of that, *disrobing*① and allowing touch—I would submit to you that that is a ritual of exceeding importance. And if you shortchange that ritual by not undressing the patient, by listening with your stethoscope on top of the night gown, by not doing a complete exam, you have bypassed on the opportunity to seal the patient-physician relationship.

20　I am a writer, and I want to close by reading you a short passage that I wrote that has to do very much with this scene. I'm an infectious disease physician, and in the early days of HIV, before we had our medications, I presided over so many scenes like this. I remember, every time I went to a patient's deathbed, whether in the hospital or at home, I remember my sense of failure—the feeling of I don't know what I have to say; I don't know what I can say; I don't know what I'm supposed to do. And out of that sense of failure, I remember, I would always examine the patient. I would pull down the eyelids. I would

吧? 我们用仪式表达权力的交接,我们用仪式标注生命的过往。仪式非常重要,它意味着改变。我想告诉你们的是,当一个人来到另一个人面前,向他／她说出一些都不曾向神父坦白的话,甚至还宽衣解带允许对方的触碰,这本就是个非常重要的仪式。如果你还在仪式的程序上偷懒,比如不解衣服、隔着睡衣听诊,或者检查不完整,你就已经错过了和病人建立良好医患关系的最佳机会。

20　我是个作家,我想以我曾写过的一段话来结束这个演讲,因为它与这个场景正契合。我是个传染病医生,在HIV治疗还没有药物干预的时候,我经常会经历这样的一幕。每每在医院或病人家的卧榻前,我常感到深深的挫败——一种无话可说,无话能说,也无力可为的挫败感。我记得,在这种挫败感之下,我唯一能做的就是检查病人——翻翻眼皮,看看舌头,敲敲胸部,听听心跳,按按腹部。很多病人,他们的名字依然萦绕耳边,他们的脸庞依

---

① disrobing *adj.* 裸露的

look at the tongue. I would percuss the chest. I would listen to the heart. I would feel the abdomen. I remember so many patients, their names still vivid on my tongue, their faces still so clear. I remember so many huge, hollowed out, haunted eyes staring up at me as I performed this ritual. And then the next day, I would come, and I would do it again.

然历历在目。在我进行这些例行的检查仪式时，那些大而空洞的眼睛，就这样茫然地看着我。第二天我还会来，重复同样的仪式。

21   And I wanted to read you this one closing passage about one patient. "I recall one patient who was at that point no more than a *skeleton*① encased in shrinking skin, unable to speak, his mouth crusted with *candida*② that was resistant to the usual medications. When he saw me on what turned out to be his last hours on this earth, his hands moved as if in slow motion. And as I wondered what he was up to, his stick fingers made their way up to his pajama shirt, fumbling with his buttons. I realized that he was wanting to expose his wicker-basket chest to me. It was an offering, an invitation. I did not decline."

21   我想给各位读的结束语，是关于一位病人的："我记起了这样一位病人，他瘦骨嶙峋，形容枯槁，已无力言语。他的嘴里长满念珠菌，这种真菌对普通药物已经产生了抗药性，因此无药可医。当他看见我时，已是他活在人世的最后几个小时。他的手如慢动作一般缓缓移动。我不知他想做什么，但当他干柴一样的手指，伸向睡衣，摸索着开始解扣子时，我意识到，他是想给我看看他骨瘦如柴的胸膛。那是个邀请，一次仪式的邀请，我没有拒绝。"

22   "I percussed. I *palpated*③. I listened to the chest. I think he surely must have known by then that it was vital for me just as it was necessary for him. Neither of us could skip this

22   "我对他进行了叩诊、触诊，也听了胸腔。我想他一定知道，这个仪式对我如此重要，正如对

---

① skeleton *n.* 骨架
② candida *n.* 念珠菌
③ palpate *v.* 触诊

ritual, which had nothing to do with detecting *rales*① in the lung, or finding the *gallop*② rhythm of heart failure. No, this ritual was about the one message that physicians have needed to convey to their patients. Although, God knows, of late, in our *hubris*③, we seem to have drifted away. We seem to have forgotten—as though, with the explosion of knowledge, the whole human *genome*④ mapped out at our feet, we are lulled into inattention, forgetting that the ritual is *cathartic*⑤ to the physician, necessary for the patient—forgetting that the ritual has meaning and a *singular*⑥ message to convey to the patient.

他也必不可少一样。谁也不能省略这个仪式，这么做不是为了听肺部的杂音，或是心脏衰弱的跳动。不，这是一个医生在向患者传达着信息。老天爷才知道，现在的我们变得有多么狂妄自大，我们似乎已经得意忘形了。知识大爆炸，人类基因组测序成功，我们被胜利冲昏了头脑。我们开始变得健忘，忘记了仪式对病人和医生有多重要，忘记了它是情感宣泄的方式，忘记了仪式的意义，也忘记了用它向病人传达那特殊的信息。"

23 "And the message, which I didn't fully understand then, even as I delivered it, and which I understand better now is this: I will always, always, always be there. I will see you through this. I will never abandon you. I will be with you through the end."

23 "当时的我并不知道那要传达的信息究竟是什么，可现在我明白了。我要告诉他的就是——我会永远守护你，永远，永远；我会陪你经历一切；我绝不会离你而去；我会陪你直到最后。"

24 Thank you very much.

24 谢谢！

---

① rale *n.* 肺的诊音
② gallop *n.* 急速，飞奔
③ hubris *n.* 骄傲，自大
④ genome *n.* 基因组，染色体组
⑤ cathartic *adj.* 精神宣泄的
⑥ singular *adj.* 奇特的，非凡的

演讲赏析

　　这是一篇成功的政策类说服性演讲（persuasive speech on questions of policy）。演讲者按照问题—出路（problem-solution）的逻辑展开论证，通过一系列生动的故事和个人经历，说明了"人文关怀"这一仪式感的重要性，呼吁医生们重新回到传统的一对一的诊断方式。

　　演讲的开头，演讲者讲述了一个故事（tell a story）：一位病人入院检查多次，竟没有被发现患有乳腺肿瘤，导致肿瘤扩展到全身。接下来，演讲者关联听众（relate to the audience），指出了一个令人担忧的现状：现代医疗对仪器过分依赖，成功吸引了听众的兴趣（arouse the interest of the audience）。然后通过提要句（preview statement）直接表明了演讲主题（topic）：医学最重要的发明就是人类之手的力量——关爱、抚慰、诊断和治疗。

　　演讲主体包括三个部分。第一部分，演讲者通过事例（examples）回忆了过去内科医生对病人的人文关怀（main point one）。演讲者讲述了柯南·道尔笔下福尔摩斯的原型——贝尔医生和病人之间的沟通，这种对话的细节描写让听众身临其境，深受触动。接下来，演讲者回顾了人类用感官诊疗疾病的历史，从拔火罐放血的内科诊疗，到叩诊法、听诊器的出现，到《医生》这幅画的内涵，为接下来的对比做好铺垫。第二部分，演讲者通过对比和叙述个人经历（personal experience）论证了人文关怀的逐步缺失（main point two）。演讲者把现在的病人比喻为"电子病人"。对"过去围绕病人"和"现在围绕电脑"两种诊疗方式进行了对比，生动说明了"*There's a real disjunction between the patient's perception and our own perceptions as physicians of the best medical care.*"演讲者还叙述了两个自己深有感触的故事，分别从病人和医生的角度（peer testimony and expert testimony）来看待人文关怀的重要性，提高了说服的可信度（credibility）。同时，演讲者有效运用了单一数据（single statistics）："*We know the average American physician interrupts their patient in 14 seconds. And if I ever get to heaven, it will be because I held my piece for 45 minutes and did not interrupt my patient.*"第三部分，演讲者从人类学的角度论证了"一对一的诊断方式"这种仪式感对病人的必要性（main point three）。

　　在演讲的结尾，演讲者通过对一位病人具体生动的描述，唤起听众的情感反应

(appealing to emotions),再次强化了演讲的主题:病人需要这种仪式的人文关怀。最后三个 always 的重复(repetition)和三个排比句(parallelism)的运用增强了情感上的共鸣,生动而有感染力,使演讲达到高潮。

本篇演讲最大的特点是大量使用例证,包括扩展例证(extended example)、简要例证(brief examples)和假设例证(hypothetical examples)。这些例证能够增强演讲的可信度,激发群众的情感共鸣,大大增加了演讲的生命力和影响力。

 精彩加油站

Got a Meeting? Take a Walk
要开会? 边走边谈

精彩视频

What you're doing, right now, at this very moment, is killing you. More than cars or the Internet or even that little mobile device we keep talking about, the technology you're using the most almost every day is this, your tush. Nowadays people are sitting 9.3 hours a day, which is more than we're sleeping, at 7.7 hours. Sitting is so incredibly prevalent, we don't even question how much we're doing it, and because everyone else is doing it, it doesn't even occur to us that it's not okay. In that way, sitting has become the smoking of our generation.

就在此时此刻,你所做的事情,正危及你的生命。我所说的是一种我们每天使用频率极高的工具,甚至比汽车、网络或是我们一直在讨论的那种小型移动设备还要高——它就是你的臀部。如今人们每天要坐 9.3 个小时,这比睡眠花费的 7.7 个小时还要长。"坐"是如此盛行,以至于我们从来都不会去质疑我们到底坐了多长时间。因为每个人都在坐着,我们也从来没觉得这有什么问题。就这样,"坐",成为我们这代人慢性自杀的方式之一,就像吸烟一样。

Of course there's health consequences to this, scary ones, besides the waist. Things like breast cancer and colon cancer are directly tied to our lack of physical inactivity. Ten percent in fact, on both of those. Six percent for heart disease, seven percent for Type Ⅱ diabetes, which is what my father died of. Now, any of those stats should convince each of us to get off our duff more, but if you're anything like me, it won't.

What did get me moving was a social interaction. Someone invited me to a meeting, but couldn't manage to fit me in to a regular sort of conference room meeting, and said, "I have to walk my dogs tomorrow. Could you come then?" It seemed kind of odd to do, and actually, that first meeting, I remember thinking, "I have to be the one to ask the next question," because I knew I was going to huff and puff during this conversation. And yet, I've taken that idea and made it my own. So instead of going to coffee meetings or fluorescent-lit conference room meetings, I ask people to go on a walking meeting, to the tune of 20 to 30 miles a week. It's changed my life.

But before that, what actually happened was, I used to think about it as, you could take care of your health, or you could take

当然，久坐带来的不仅仅是腰围的增加，它还会引发许多可怕的健康问题。乳癌和大肠癌都与长时间不运动紧密相关。事实上，以上两种疾病的患病率都因久坐不动增长了 10%。心脏病的患病率因此增长了 6%，而我父亲的致命病因——二型糖尿病的患病率也因此增加了 7%。现在，这些数据应该能说服我们每个人站起身来动一动屁股了吧？但如果你和我是同一类人，你还是不会动。

真正让我动起来的是一次社交活动。有人邀请我去参加一个会议，但却没办法安排我去常规的会议室，于是他说："明天我要去遛狗。你方便那时候来吗？"这听上去有些怪异，事实上，记得首次进行这种会议的时候，我一直在想："接下来的问题得由我来问"，因为我知道我马上就只能气喘吁吁地说话了。但是，我接受了这个点子并使之成为我的点子。我不再边喝咖啡边开会，也不再去灯光闪亮的会议室开会，而是邀请人们进行散步会议，平均每周走 20 到 30 英里。这改变了我的生活。

但在此之前的实际情况是，我曾认为，你要么能照顾好自己的身体，要么能履行好自己的职责，想要

care of obligations, and one always came at the cost of the other. So now, several hundred of these walking meetings later, I've learned a few things.

First, there's this amazing thing about actually getting out of the box that leads to out-of-the-box thinking. Whether it's nature or the exercise itself, it certainly works.

And second, and probably the more reflective one, is just about how much each of us can hold problems in opposition when they're really not that way. And if we're going to solve problems and look at the world really differently, whether it's in governance or business or environmental issues, job creation, maybe we can think about how to reframe those problems as having both things be true. Because it was when that happened with this walk-and-talk idea that things became doable and sustainable and viable.

So I started this talk talking about the tush, so I'll end with the bottom line, which is, walk and talk. Walk the talk. You'll be surprised at how fresh air drives fresh thinking, and in the way that you do, you'll bring into your life an entirely new set of ideas.

Thank you.

实现其一，总是以牺牲另一方为代价的。因此，在开展了几百次散步会议之后，我学到了一些东西。

首先，能够从固有框架中跳出来，思维不再墨守成规，的确是一件令人惊喜的事情。不管这是因为大自然还是锻炼本身的原因，效果的确存在。

其次，也许更让人深思的是，我们是否能够将对立的问题兼容考虑，当问题本身并非如此的时候。假如我们打算去解决问题，并换一种方式来看待世界的话，不管是政府问题、商业问题、环境问题还是就业问题，也许我们可以考虑跳出这些问题的框架，兼顾所有的需求。因为正是有了这种边走边谈的想法，才使一切变得可行。

我以"臀部"作为演说的开端，也将以此来收尾：边走边谈，边谈边走。你会惊讶地发现新鲜的空气能激发创新的思维。只要你坚持这样做，一套崭新的观点将会融入你的生活。

谢谢。

Lecture 2　What You Need To Know About Ebola

你们需要了解的关于埃博拉的事情

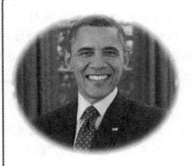

　　美国总统有个传统，就是每周六都要做一个电台演讲。历史上最著名的总统电台演讲是 20 世纪 30—40 年代美国经济大萧条时期，罗斯福总统的"炉边谈话"（fireside chats）。不过直到里根总统时代，才正式成为每个星期的惯例，第一次的每周电台演讲（weekly radio address）是在 1982 年 4 月 3 日。一个短小的演讲，却能拉近一个国家最有权力的人和平民百姓间的距离。今天跟大家分享的是美国前总统奥巴马在 2014 年 10 月 18 日做的电视演讲，他同康复的埃博拉患者在椭圆形办公室会面，主要跟民众讲了关于埃博拉的一些常识。奥式口音，衬衫领带，职业演讲家奥巴马亲自上阵，为你主播美国版"新闻联播"。

1 Today, I want to take a few minutes, to speak with you—directly and clearly—about *Ebola*①, what we're doing about it, and what you need to know, because meeting a public health challenge like this isn't just a job for government. All of us—citizens, leaders, the media—have a responsibility and a role to play. This is a serious disease, but we can't give in to *hysteria*② or fear, because that only makes it harder to get people the accurate information they need. We have to be guided by the science. We have to remember the basic facts.

2 First, what we're seeing now is not an "outbreak" or an "*epidemic*③" of Ebola in America. We're a nation of more than 300 million people. To date, we've seen three cases of Ebola *diagnosed*④ here: the man who *contracted*⑤ the disease in *Liberia*⑥, came here and sadly died; the two courageous nurses who were infected while they were treating him. Our thoughts and our prayers are with them, and we're doing everything we can to give them the best care possible. Now, even one

1　今天，我想花几分钟的时间，直接和明确地与你们谈谈埃博拉，包括我们目前针对它所采取的措施，以及一些你们需要了解的事情，因为处理一个这样的公共卫生挑战，不仅仅是政府的工作，我们所有人——公民、领袖、媒体——都有责任，各司其职。埃博拉是一种很严重的疾病，但我们不能任由这种抓狂或是恐慌的情绪控制我们，因为这样只会让人们更难得到他们需要的准确信息。我们必须以科学为指导。我们必须记住一些基本的事实。

2　首先，我们现在在美国见到的并不是埃博拉病毒的"爆发"或者"疫情"。我们是一个拥有超过3亿国民的国家。到目前为止，我们知道被诊断为埃博拉的病例只有3个：一例是在利比里亚感染了病毒的男性，到美国后不幸去世；另外两例都是勇敢的护士，在为其治疗时被感染。我们为她们担心，为她们祈祷，我们也正在尽我们所能给予她们最好的治

① Ebola *n.* 埃博拉病毒
② hysteria *n.* 歇斯底里
③ epidemic *n.* 传染病；流行病
④ diagnose *v.* 诊断
⑤ contract *v.* 感染
⑥ Liberia *n.* 利比里亚（西非）

*infection*① is too many. At the same time, we have to keep this in perspective. As our public health experts point out, every year thousands of Americans die from the flu.

现疗。现在,哪怕再多一个病例我们也不想看到。可与此同时,我们也必须客观地看待这个问题。正如我们的公共卫生专家所指出的那样,每年还有成千上万的美国人会死于流感。

3　Second, Ebola is actually a difficult disease to catch. It's not *transmitted*② through the air like the flu. You cannot get it from just riding on a plane or a bus. The only way that a person can contract the disease is by coming into direct contact with the *bodily fluids*③ of somebody who is already showing *symptoms*④. I've met and hugged some of the doctors and nurses who've treated Ebola patients. I've met with an Ebola patient who recovered right in the Oval Office. And I'm fine.

3　第二,埃博拉实际上是一种很难传播的疾病。它并不会像流感那样通过空气传播。仅仅是乘坐飞机或者坐公交车,你是不会被感染的。能够感染这一病毒的唯一方式是直接接触到已经出现症状的患者体液。我已经见过了治疗埃博拉患者的医生和护士,并和他们进行拥抱。我也在白宫总统办公室会见了一名埃博拉患者。我现在没有任何问题。

4　Third, we know how to fight this disease, we know the *protocols*⑤. And we know that when they're followed, they work. So far, five Americans who got infected with Ebola in West Africa have been brought back to the United States, and all five have been treated safely, without infecting healthcare workers. And this

4　第三,我们知道该如何应对这一疾病,我们知道治疗方案。我们明白,只要遵循这些方案,它们就可以用来抗击埃博拉。到目前为止,五名在西非感染了埃博拉的国人,已经被带回国内,五个人都得到了安全治疗,也没有医

---

① infection *n.* 感染;传染
② transmit *v.* 传播
③ bodily fluids 体液
④ symptom *n.* 症状
⑤ protocol *n.* 医疗方案

week, at my direction, we're stepping up our efforts. Additional **CDC**① personnel are on the scene in Dallas and Cleveland. We're working quickly to track and monitor anyone who may have been in close contact with someone showing symptoms. We're sharing lessons learned, so other hospitals don't repeat the mistakes that happened in Dallas. The CDC's new Ebola rapid response teams will deploy quickly to help hospitals implement the right protocols. New *screening*② measures are now in place at airports that receive nearly all passengers arriving from Liberia, *Guinea*③ and *Sierra Leone*④. And we'll continue to constantly review our measures and update them as needed, to make sure we're doing everything we can to keep Americans safe.

5　Finally, we can't just cut ourselves off from West Africa where this disease is *raging*⑤. Our medical experts tell us that the best way to stop this disease is to stop it at its source, before it spreads even wider and becomes even more difficult to contain. Trying to seal off an entire region of the world, if that were even possible,

护人员被感染。本周,在我的指示下,各项工作正紧锣密鼓地展开。疾控中心派出更多人手在达拉斯和克利夫兰的现场工作。我们正在快速地追踪和监测任何可能与出现症状的患者有密切接触的人。我们也在分享经验教训,以便其他医院不会重复在达拉斯犯过的错误。疾控中心新的快速反应小组可以迅速部署,以协助各医院实施正确的治疗方案。在机场,新的筛查措施已经开始实施,几乎所有来自利比里亚、几内亚和塞拉利昂的乘客都将接受检查。我们将继续不断审查我们的措施,并根据需要进行修改,以确保我们能尽一切努力来保护国人的安全。

5　最后,我们不能仅仅阻断与疫情正在肆虐的西非的联系。我们的医疗专家指出,控制这一疾病的最好方式,是在它蔓延更广、变得更难控制之前,在源头上阻止它。即便封锁某个地区的做法是可行的,但实际上只能让形势更加恶化。这将使医疗工作者和

---

① CDC Center for Disease Control (美国)疾病控制中心
② screening *n.* 筛查
③ Guinea 几内亚(西非)
④ Sierra Leone 塞拉利昂(西非)
⑤ rage *v.* (灾、病等的)猖獗;肆虐

could actually make the situation worse. It would make it harder to move health workers and supplies back and forth. Experience shows that it could also cause people in the affected region to change their travel, to evade screening, and make the disease even harder to track. So the United States will continue to help lead the global response in West Africa. Because if we want to protect Americans from Ebola here at home, we have to end it over there. And as our civilian and military personnel serve in the region, their safety and health will remain a top priority.

6　As I've said before, fighting this disease will take time. Before this is over, we may see more isolated cases here in America, but we know how to wage this fight. And if we take the steps that are necessary, if we're guided by the science—the facts, not fear, then I am absolutely confident that we can prevent a serious outbreak here in the United States, and we can continue to lead the world in this urgent effort.

物资的往来变得更加困难。经验表明，这也会导致受感染地区的人们改变行程，逃避筛查，最终使疾病变得更加难以追踪。因此，美国将继续在西非开展的埃博拉疫情全球应对工作中扮演重要角色，因为如果我们想看到疫情在国内终结，西非将是第一步。只要我们有国人和士兵在那里工作，保障他们的安全与健康将一直是我们工作的重中之重。

6　正如我之前所说，战胜这一疾病需要时间。在一切结束之前，我们可能会在美国看到更多的单个病例，但我们知道如何进行这场战斗。如果我们采取必要的步骤，如果我们遵循科学——遵循事实，而不是恐惧，那么我绝对有信心说，我们可以避免埃博拉病毒在美国的严重爆发，我们也能够继续引领全球为完成这一迫切任务而努力。

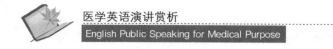
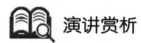 演讲赏析

2014 年,西非埃博拉病毒爆发,规模之大史无前例,并蔓延到其他国家和地区。美国的两名医务人员在参与治疗美国本土首名埃博拉确诊患者后感染病毒。美国作为一个高医疗水平的国家,在应对埃博拉的防线中出现如此漏洞,使得不少医疗专家和媒体开始产生怀疑。加上恐惧和错误信息,很多美国民众也开始担心疫情在本土扩散。

在这样的背景下,总统的这次每周演讲起到了传播知识、共享信息的作用,不煽情、不喊口号,而是直接明白地告知美国人需要知道的关键事实,属于典型的说解性演讲(informative speech)。整篇演讲结构清晰、语言平实,易于理解和接受。

这篇演讲从标题(title)"What You Need To Know About Ebola"开始就直插主题,把演讲内容的核心简明地提示出来,不含蓄、不抒情也不抽象。在当时的局势下,直接和明确就是最好的方式。

开篇语(introduction)部分简明扼要,奥巴马的第一句话(Today, I want to take a few minutes, to speak with you—directly and clearly—about Ebola, what we're doing about it, and what you need to know.)就是一个提要句(preview statement),明确地告知大家他今天要讲的主要内容和目的,然后又通过几句话阐明了他这个演讲的重要性,引起听众的注意。

然后在主体内容(body)部分,他从四个方面讨论了埃博拉病毒:第一,在美国见到的并不是埃博拉疾病的爆发或疫情;第二,感染这一病毒的唯一方式是直接接触到已有患者的体液;第三,人们已经知道该如何应对这一疾病;最后,他表示控制这一疾病的最好方式是在源头上制止它。这四个要点(main points)按照话题顺序法(topical order)进行组织,层层递进、逻辑性强,并使用了 First, Second 等数字作为提示语(signpost),条理清晰。在说明事实时,用了具体的数据(statistics)、专家的证言(testimony)以及他本人的经历(example)等辅助资料(supporting idea)来增加可信度,又不乏人情味。总统本人并非医疗专家,大部分民众也只是普通人,所以这部分内容虽然涉及疾病,但都浅显易懂。

最后,在结束语(conclusion)中,奥巴马总统明确表示,他和他的政府将继续尽一切努力,防止疾病在国内进一步传播,并引领全球对抗埃博拉疫情。这段内容和开篇语首尾呼应,重申了主题和要点,深化了听众对这次演讲内容的理解。

同时我们也能注意到,虽然这是一篇说解性的演讲,但是奥巴马作为总统,掌握大局、思路清晰,整个演讲显得充满自信,也起到了安慰民心、避免恐慌的作用。

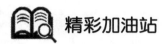 **精彩加油站**

Why Genetic Research Must Be More Diverse
人类基因研究需要更多样化

精彩视频

As a little Hawaiian, my mom and auntie always told me stories about Kalaupapa—the Hawaiian leper colony surrounded by the highest sea cliffs in the world—and Father Damien, the Belgian missionary who gave his life for the Hawaiian community. As a young nurse, my aunt trained the nuns caring for the remaining lepers almost 100 years after Father Damien died of leprosy. I remember stories she told about traveling down switchback cliff paths on a mule, while my uncle played her favorite hula songs on the ukulele all the way down to Kalaupapa.

You see, as a youngster, I was always curious about a few things. First was why a Belgian missionary chose to live in complete isolation in Kalaupapa, knowing he would

我是夏威夷人,在我很小的时候,我的母亲和姑姑总是跟我讲卡劳帕帕半岛的故事。那是夏威夷的麻风病人隔离区,被世界上最高的海崖包围着。她们还会讲到一位名叫达米安的比利时传教士,他为这个社区献出了自己的生命。在达米安传教士因麻风病逝世近一百年后,我的姑姑,一名年轻的护士,教修女们照顾那里剩下的麻风病人。我依旧记得她讲的故事:她和我的叔叔骑着骡子穿行在陡峭的悬崖小路上,叔叔用尤克里里琴弹奏她最喜欢的草裙舞曲,就这样一路来到卡劳帕帕。

那时的我一直对一些事感到好奇。首先,为什么一个比利时传教士选择在卡劳帕帕过着与世隔绝的生活?他明明知道帮助这些病人,

inevitably contract leprosy from the community of people he sought to help. And secondly, where did the leprosy bacteria come from? And why were Kānaka Maoli, the indigenous people of Hawaii, so susceptible to developing leprosy, or "mai Pake?"

This got my curious about what makes us unique as Hawaiians—namely, our genetic makeup. But it wasn't until high school, through the Human Genome Project, that I realized I wasn't alone in trying to connect our unique genetic ancestry to our potential health, wellness and illness. You see, the 2.7 billion-dollar project promised an era of predictive and preventative medicine based on our unique genetic makeup. So to me it always seemed obvious that in order to achieve this dream, we would need to sequence a diverse cohort of people to obtain the full spectrum of human genetic variation on the planet. That's why 10 years later, it continues to shock me, knowing that 96 percent of genome studies associating common genetic variation with specific diseases have focused exclusively on individuals of European ancestry.

Now you don't need a PhD to see that that leaves four percent for the rest of diversity. And in my own searching, I've discovered that far less than one percent have

就会不可避免地传染上麻风病。还有，卡劳帕帕半岛的麻风病菌是从哪里来的？为什么夏威夷的土著居民会特别容易感染麻风病（夏威夷语称之为 mai Pake）？

这一切都让我好奇，是什么让我们夏威夷人与众不同？换句话说，我们的基因构成究竟有什么特别的地方？我直到高中参加了一个人类基因组的项目后，才意识到我并不是唯一一个试图将我们独特的遗传基因与身体潜在的患病概率联系起来的人。要知道，这个耗资27亿美元的计划可是有希望让我们通过研究特有的基因组成，把人类引入一个疾病可预测、可预防的新医疗时代的。对我而言，要完成这样一个梦想，我们需要对不同群体进行基因测序，以获得人类基因遗传变异全谱，这是再明显不过的了。这也是为什么十年过去了，有一个现状仍然让我感到震惊——为特定疾病与常见基因变异建立关联的基因研究中，有96%仍然是以欧裔人为唯一研究对象的。

即使没有博士学位的人都能看出来，对其他种族的基因研究只占到4%。在我自己的研究项目里，针对像我一样的土著居民的研究远

actually focused on indigenous communities，like myself. So that begs the question：Who is the Human Genome Project actually for? Just like we have different colored eyes and hair，we metabolize drugs differently based on the variation in our genomes. So how many of you would be shocked to learn that 95 percent of clinical trials have also exclusively featured individuals of European ancestry?

This bias and systematic lack of engagement of indigenous people in both clinical trials and genome studies is partially the result of a history of distrust. For example，in 1989，researchers from Arizona State University obtained blood samples from Arizona's Havasupai tribe，promising to alleviate the burden of type 2 diabetes that was plaguing their community，only to turn around and use those exact same samples—without the Havasupai's consent—to study rates of schizophrenia，inbreeding，and challenge the Havasupai's origin story. When the Havasupai found out，they sued successfully for ＄700,000，and they banned ASU from conducting research on their reservation. This culminated in a sort of domino effect with local tribes in the Southwest—including the Navajo Nation，one of the largest tribes in the country—putting a moratorium on genetic research.

不到 1%。所以我要问一个问题：人类基因组计划究竟是为了谁？正如我们有着不同颜色的眼睛和头发，我们对药物的代谢能力也会因基因组的差异而有所不同。那么当你们知道 95% 的药物临床试验也是针对欧裔人群时，你们当中又有多少人会感到震惊呢？

临床试验和基因组研究中的种族偏见以及土著居民的长期参与缺席，部分源于双方在历史上的信任危机。举个例子，1989 年，亚利桑那州州立大学的研究人员在亚利桑那州哈瓦苏部落采集了血样，并承诺该研究将降低困扰当地居民的 2 型糖尿病的发生率。不料，在没有经过哈瓦苏人同意的情况下，研究者竟然用这些血样来分析精神分裂症和近亲繁殖的概率，并且质疑了哈瓦苏部落的起源。当哈瓦苏人获悉事情真相后，他们发起诉讼并成功获赔 70 万美元，同时禁止亚利桑那州州立大学对其部落进行研究。这件事在美国西南部造成了多米诺效应。当地的部落，包括美国最大的部落纳瓦霍族，都叫停了基因研究。

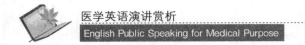

Now despite this history of distrust, I still believe that indigenous people can benefit from genetic research. And if we don't do something soon, the gap in health disparities is going to continue to widen. Hawaii, for example, has the longest life expectancy on average of any state in the US, yet native Hawaiians like myself die a full decade before our non-native counterparts, because we have some of the highest rates of type 2 diabetes, obesity, and the number one and number two killers in the US: cardiovascular disease and cancer.

So how do we ensure the populations of people that need genome sequencing the most are not the last to benefit? My vision is to make genetic research more native, to indigenize genome sequencing technology.

Traditionally, genomes are sequenced in laboratories. Here's an image of your classic genome sequencer. It's huge. It's the size of a refrigerator. There's this obvious physical limitation. But what if you could sequence genomes on the fly? What if you could fit a genome sequencer in your pocket? This nanopore-based sequencer is one 10,000th the size of your traditional genome sequencer. It doesn't have the same physical limitations, in that it's not tethered to a lab bench with extraneous cords, large vats of chemicals or computer monitors. It allows us to de-black

尽管有这段不信任的历史,我仍然相信,土著居民能够从基因研究中获益。如果我们不尽快采取行动,医疗健康的差距将继续扩大。以夏威夷为例,在美国所有州中,夏威夷人是平均寿命最长的。但是像我这样的夏威夷原住民,比非原住民的寿命要短整整十年。因为我们的2型糖尿病、肥胖症、心血管疾病和癌症的发病率最高,其中心血管疾病和癌症同时也是美国人健康的头号和二号杀手。

那么,对于最需要检测基因组序列的人群,我们该如何确保他们的利益呢?我的想法是基因研究和基因测序技术都可以进一步本土化。

一般来说,基因组测序是在实验室中进行的。这是一张传统的基因序列测定仪的照片。它很大,有一个冰箱大小。很明显,它对使用环境有一定限制。但如果你能在飞行途中测序呢?如果你能用口袋装下一个基因序列测定仪呢?这个纳米孔测序仪只有传统测定仪的万分之一大小。它对使用环境没有限制,因为它不需要被固定在实验室的工作台上,它也没有多余的数据线、大量的化学药品或显示器。它使我们能够以融入和合作的方法解

box genome sequencing technology development in a way that's immersive and collaborative, activating and empowering indigenous communities ... as citizen scientists.

100 years later in Kalaupapa, we now have the technology to sequence leprosy bacteria in real time, using mobile genome sequencers, remote access to the Internet and cloud computation. But only if that's what Hawaiian people want. In our space, on our terms.

IndiGenomics is about science for the people by the people. We'll be starting with a tribal consultation resource, focused on educating indigenous communities on the potential use and misuse of genetic information. Eventually we'd like to have our own IndiGenomics research institute to conduct our own experiments and educate the next generation of indigenous scientists.

In the end, indigenous people need to be partners in and not subjects of genetic research. And for those on the outside, just as Father Damien did, the research community needs to immerse itself in indigenous culture or die trying.

Mahalo.

密基因测序技术的发展，让土著居民有动力和能力研究基因序列，使他们成为公民科学家。

一百年之后，在卡劳帕帕，移动基因测序仪的使用，互联网访问和云计算的实现，使实时测序麻风细菌的技术已成为现实。当然前提是这是我们夏威夷人的意愿——在我们的地方，按我们的规矩来。

本土基因学应该是人民的科学。我们会从部落咨询会开始，重点告诉本土居民对于基因信息的正当和不正当使用。最终，我们想要成立自己本土的基因研究机构来进行我们自己的研究，也要培养下一代的本土科学家。

最后，我要说的是，本土居民应该成为基因研究的成员，而不是基因研究的对象。那些非本土的研究团队，则应该像达米安神父那样，让自己更多地融入土著文化中，并不顾一切地去尝试。

谢谢！（夏威夷语）

Lecture 3   The Brain May Be Able to Repair Itself—With Help

大脑也许可以在辅助下进行自我修复

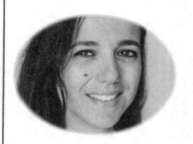

　　乔斯林·布洛赫（Jocelyne Bloch），瑞士神经外科医生，洛桑大学医院（CHUV）功能神经科主任，是通过深部脑刺激和神经调节来治疗运动障碍疾病的专家。她目前重点研究与神经形成和大脑修复相关的皮层细胞，即双皮质素。与让·弗朗索瓦·布鲁内特（Jean François Brunet）及其他研究人员共同合作，首创了利用中风病人自身的细胞进行大脑细胞移植的治疗方法。她致力于将所有的创新式治疗方法进行收集汇总，以便为神经损伤的病人提供最佳治疗方案。

1　So I'm a *neurosurgeon*①. And like most of my colleagues, I have to deal, every day, with human tragedies. I realize how your life can change from one second to the other after a major stroke or after a car accident. And what is very frustrating for us neurosurgeons is to realize that unlike other organs of the body, the brain has very little ability for self-repair. And after a major injury of your central nervous system, the patients often remain with a severe handicap. And that's probably the reason why I've chosen to be a functional neurosurgeon.

2　What is a functional neurosurgeon? It's a doctor who is trying to improve a neurological function through different surgical strategies. You've certainly heard of one of the famous ones called deep brain stimulation, where you *implant*② an *electrode*③ in the depths of the brain in order to *modulate*④ a circuit of neurons to improve a neurological function. It's really an amazing technology in that it has improved the destiny of patients with Parkinson's disease, with severe *tremor*⑤, with severe pain. However, neuromodulation does not mean neuro-repair. And the dream of functional neurosurgeons is to repair the brain. I think

1　我是一名神经外科医生。就像我的大部分同事一样，我每天要面对很多人间悲剧。这让我明白，人可能因为一次严重的中风或车祸而瞬间改变一生的命运。而最令我们这些神经外科医生苦恼的，就是知道大脑不像其他器官，它很难自我修复。如果中枢神经系统受到严重损伤，患者常常会面临终身残疾。这可能也是我想要成为一名功能神经外科医生的原因。

2　功能神经外科医生是做什么工作的呢？他们通过不同的手术方法来改善神经功能。你们一定听过其中一个著名的方法叫做深度脑部刺激，就是把一个电极植入大脑深处，通过调控神经元电流来改善神经功能。这项技术不可思议地扭转了患有帕金森症，被震颤和剧痛困扰的病人的命运。但是，神经调控并不意味着神经元的修复。功能神经外科医生希望有朝一日能够修复受损的大脑。我想，我们正在一步一步接近这个目标。

① neurosurgeon *n.* 神经外科医生
② implant *v.* 移植
③ electrode *n.* 电极
④ modulate *v.* 调节
⑤ tremor *n.* 震颤

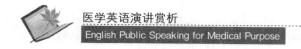

that we are approaching this dream.

3　And I would like to show you that we are very close to this; and that with a little bit of help, the brain is able to help itself.

4　So the story started 15 years ago. At that time, I was a chief resident working days and nights in the emergency room. I often had to take care of patients with head *trauma*①. You have to imagine that when a patient comes in with a severe head trauma, his brain is *swelling*② and he's increasing his *intracranial*③ pressure. And in order to save his life, you have to decrease this intracranial pressure. And to do that, you sometimes have to remove a piece of swollen brain. So instead of throwing away these pieces of swollen brain, we decided with Jean-François Brunet, who is a colleague of mine, a biologist, to study them.

5　What do I mean by that? We wanted to grow cells from these pieces of tissue. It's not an easy task. Growing cells from a piece of tissue is a bit the same as growing very small children out

3　而且,我想告诉大家,我们离成功已经近在咫尺了,我们发现只需要一点点的人工辅助,大脑其实是可以进行自我修复的。

4　事情还要从 15 年前说起。那时候我还是一名住院总医师,夜以继日地在急诊室忙碌。我经常需要救治大脑受到损伤的病患。你们可以想象出那是什么样的情景。一位严重的脑外伤患者入院时,大脑不断肿胀,颅内压越来越高。这时要挽救他的生命,就必须降低颅内压。所以有时候就需要移除一部分肿胀的脑组织。不过我们并没有把这一部分脑组织直接丢弃,而是决定和我的同事,生物学家让·弗朗索瓦·布鲁内特对这些组织进行进一步的研究。

5　具体要怎么研究呢? 我们想从这些脑组织中培育细胞。可这并非易事。从一块脑组织培育细胞,就类似离开了父母来抚育小

---

①　trauma *n.* 创伤,外伤
②　swell *v.* 肿胀,肿大(swelled, swollen)
③　intracranial *adj.* 颅内的

from their family. So you need to find the right nutrients, the warmth, the humidity and all the nice environments to make them thrive. So that's exactly what we had to do with these cells. And after many attempts, Jean-François did it. And that's what he saw under his microscope.

宝宝,需要找到的是合适的营养成分,适宜的温度和湿度,以保证他们能够在适宜的环境下存活。我们就是要在这样的条件下培养这些细胞。在很多次的试验之后,让·弗朗索瓦终于成功了。这就是他在显微镜下看到的一幕。

6   And that was, for us, a major surprise. Why? Because this looks exactly the same as a *stem cell*① culture, with large green cells surrounding small, immature cells. And you may remember from biology class that stem cells are immature cells, able to turn into any type of cells of the body. The adult brain has stem cells, but they're very rare and they're located in deep and small niches in the depths of the brain. So it was surprising to get this kind of stem cell culture from the superficial part of swollen brain we had in the operating theater.

6   对我们来说,这是个天大的惊喜。为什么呢? 因为这看起来跟干细胞群落几乎一模一样,尚未成熟的小细胞被一大群绿色的大细胞包围着。你们可能还记得生物课上讲过,干细胞是未发育成熟的细胞,可以演变成人体的任何一种细胞。成年人的大脑也有干细胞,只是数量很少,而且分布于大脑深处隐蔽的角落里。所以能够从手术室病人肿胀的大脑表面获得这种干细胞群落,真是太让人意外了。

7   And there was another *intriguing*② observation: Regular stem cells are very active cells—cells that divide, divide, divide very quickly. And they never die, they're immortal cells. But these cells behave differently. They

7   我们还观察到了另外一个有趣的现象:正常的干细胞非常活跃——它们不停地分裂,分裂,再分裂,非常迅速。它们永远不会死亡,能够一直存活。但是这些

---

① stem cell *n.* 干细胞
② intriguing *adj.* 有趣的

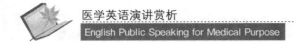

divide slowly, and after a few weeks of culture, they even died. So we were in front of a strange new cell population that looked like stem cells but behaved differently.

细胞却有着不同的表现。它们分裂得很慢，而且在几个星期的培养之后，竟然死掉了。因而我们面对的是一群奇怪的新细胞群落，看起来像干细胞，但其表现却又跟干细胞有着天壤之别。

8   And it took us a long time to understand where they came from. They come from these cells. These blue and red cells are called *doublecortin*①-positive cells. All of you have them in your brain. They represent four percent of your cortical brain cells. They have a very important role during the development stage. When you were *fetuses*②, they helped your brain to fold itself. But why do they stay in your head? This, we don't know. We think that they may participate in brain repair because we find them in higher concentration close to brain *lesions*③. But it's not so sure. But there is one clear thing—that from these cells, we got our stem cell culture. And we were in front of a potential new source of cells to repair the brain. And we had to prove this.

8   我们花了好长时间才搞清楚它们是从哪儿来的。它们来自于这些细胞。这些蓝色和红色的细胞称为双皮质素阳性细胞。它们存在于我们每个人的大脑中，组成了我们4%的大脑皮层细胞。在大脑发育过程中，这些细胞起着至关重要的作用。在胚胎期，它们帮助大脑产生褶皱。但它们为什么会一直留在大脑中呢？这一点我们还不清楚。我们认为它们可能参与了大脑修复，因为我们发现在靠近大脑损伤部位的地方，它们的浓度比较高。虽然我们还不是非常确定。但有一点已经很清楚了——也就是从这些细胞中，我们可以培养出干细胞。我们面前正是一群有可能修复大脑的新细胞。我们一定要证明这一点。

---

① doublecortin *n.* 双皮质素
② fetus *n.* 胎儿
③ lesion *n.* 损伤

9   So to prove it, we decided to design an experimental paradigm. The idea was to *biopsy*① a piece of brain in a non-eloquent area of the brain, and then to culture the cells exactly the way Jean-François did it in his lab. And then label them, to put color in them in order to be able to track them in the brain. And the last step was to re-implant them in the same individual. We call these autologous grafts—*autografts*②.

9   为了证实这一结果,我们决定设计一组实验范式。我们的基本想法就是在大脑中一块功能尚不明确的区域进行活组织提取,然后培养这些细胞,用的就是和让·弗朗索瓦在实验室里一样的操作。接着我们给它们标记、染色,以便追踪它们在大脑中的活动。最后把它们再次植入到同一个体中。我们把这种同源移植称为自体移植。

10   So the first question we had, "What will happen if we re-implant these cells in a normal brain, and what will happen if we re-implant the same cells in a lesioned brain?" Thanks to the help of professor Eric Rouiller, we worked with monkeys.

10   我们的第一个疑问就是,"如果我们把这些细胞再次植入正常的大脑,会是什么结果呢? 如果植入的是受过损伤的大脑,结果又会有什么不同?"很幸运,在埃里克·鲁耶教授的帮助下,我们得以在猴子身上进行试验。

11   So in the first-case scenario, we re-implanted the cells in the normal brain and what we saw is that they completely disappeared after a few weeks, as if they were taken from the brain, they go back home, the space is already busy, they are not needed there, so they disappear.

11   在第一种情况中,我们把这些细胞植入了正常大脑中,发现它们在仅仅几周后就完全消失了。就像是被从大脑中清除了一样,它们被驱赶出了这一区域。这里没有多余的空间了,它们发挥不了任何作用,于是就消失了。

----

① biopsy *n. & v.* 活组织提取切片检查
② autografts *n.* 自体移植术

12　　In the second-case scenario，we performed the lesion，we re-implanted exactly the same cells，and in this case，the cells remained—and they became mature neurons. And that's the image of what we could observe under the microscope. Those are the cells that were re-implanted. And the proof they carry，these little spots，those are the cells that we've labeled in vitro，when they were in culture.

13　　But we could not stop here，of course. Do these cells also help a monkey to recover after a lesion? So for that，we trained monkeys to perform a manual *dexterity*① task. They had to retrieve food pellets from a tray. They were very good at it. And when they had reached a plateau of performance，we did a lesion in the motor cortex corresponding to the hand motion. So the monkeys were plegic，they could not move their hand anymore. And exactly the same as humans would do，they spontaneously recovered to a certain extent，exactly the same as after a stroke. Patients are completely plegic，and then they try to recover due to a brain plasticity mechanism，they recover to a certain extent，exactly the same for the monkey.

14　　So when we were sure that the monkey had

12　在第二种情况中，我们用了受损的大脑，把一模一样的细胞移植进去，而这一次，细胞存活了下来——它们发育成了成熟的神经细胞。这就是我们在显微镜下看到的图像。这些是重新移植过的细胞。你看到的这些小亮点就是，因为我们当时在体外进行细胞培养时给它们做过标记。

13　但这肯定还远远不够。那么这些细胞到底能不能修复猴子的脑损伤呢？为了证明这一点，我们训练猴子完成一些需要手部灵巧度的任务。它们需要从盘子里取出小块食物。它们一向很擅长这种事儿。当它们的表现稳定后，我们在大脑的运动皮层里管理手部动作的区域人为制造了一些损伤。于是猴子们失去了手部行动能力，手再也不听使唤了。一段时间之后，它们的行动能力有了一定程度的恢复，这和人类中风后的情形类似。中风患者一开始也完全不具备行动能力，但之后会利用大脑的弹性机制会自动恢复到一定程度，猴子也是这样的。

14　于是等到我们确定猴子的自

---

① dexterity *n*. 灵巧，敏捷

reached his plateau of spontaneous recovery, we implanted his own cells. So on the left side, you see the monkey that has spontaneously recovered. He's at about 40 to 50 percent of his previous performance before the lesion. He's not so accurate, not so quick. And look now when we re-implant the cells: Two months after re-implantation, the same individual.

我恢复能力已经到达极限时，我们移植了它自身的细胞。在左边，你们可以看到猴子自行恢复的状况。与大脑受损之前的状况相比，它大概恢复了40%～50%的行动能力。它的动作不是很精准，也比较慢。再看看经过细胞移植后现在的情况：这是同一只猴子，手术后两个月。

15   It was also very exciting results for us, I tell you. Since that time, we've understood much more about these cells. We know that we can *cryopreserve*① them, we can use them later on. We know that we can apply them in other *neuropathological*② models, like Parkinson's disease, for example. But our dream is still to implant them in humans. And I really hope that I'll be able to show you soon that the human brain is giving us the tools to repair itself.

15   说实话，这样的结果就连我们也感到很意外。之后，我们对这些细胞就更加了解了。我们知道可以把这些细胞超低温冷冻，留待日后再用。我们也知道可以把它们应用到其他神经病理学病症中，比如帕金森症。但我们始终梦想有一天能把它们移植入人脑中。我真的希望很快就能让你们看到，人类大脑自我修复的工具其实一直都有，它就存在于我们的大脑里。

16   Thank you!

16   谢谢大家！

---

① cryopreserve *v.* 低温贮藏（活组织）
② neuropathological *adj.* 神经病理学的

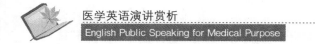

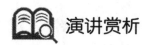 演讲赏析

　　这篇演讲属于说解性演讲（informative speech），主要向听众展示了通过实验发现大脑可以借助人为介入进行自我修复的研究结果。

　　演讲开头，演讲者首先提到了自己的身份，一名神经外科医生（neurosurgeon），这是一个好的演讲开头（introduction）中非常重要的一环，因为只有建立了信誉度（establish credibility），才能在后面的演讲中增加自己信息的可信度。另一方面，演讲者在第一和第二段中直截了当地提到了神经外科医生所面临的最大难题——大脑不像其他器官具有自我修复的功能，以及目前技术的限制。这为后面突出她的演讲话题的重要性（state the importance of your topic）做了很好的铺垫，也让听众有更大的好奇心去了解这一突破性的研究内容。

　　整篇演讲内容按照时间顺序（chronological order）展开。从一开始一次偶然的机会对脑组织细胞进行培育，到发现一种和干细胞非常类似的新细胞，再到后来为了验证他们的猜想，把这种细胞植入猴子脑内，以及最后看到的实验结果，这样的展开顺序可以让听众清楚地了解这一新的技术的内容和意义。

　　在整个演讲中，虽然介绍的是自己的科研成果，但演讲者也没有一直以 I 或者we 作为整个演讲的中心。她很好地考虑到了听众的感受，通过关联听众（relate the topic to the audience）的方式让他们可以更好地融入演讲中来。例如第一段中提到车祸和中风对大脑的损伤，以及第六段提到每个听众在生物课上都会了解到什么是干细胞。这样的表达方式可以让听众产生亲切感，使演讲更接近于一场演讲者与听众的对话（conversation）。另外，演讲者在语言上也注意了生动性，避免使用过于专业的表达，影响普通听众对这些专业知识的理解。例如第五段中在说到培养脑组织细胞时，她借用了一个明喻（simile），把这个过程生动地比喻成培养孩子。而在她必须涉及专业词汇时，她也尽量用通俗的语言进行解释，例如第九段中，她先说到 *to re-implant them in the same individual*，然后才提到自体移植（autografts）这一专业词汇。

　　在演讲的演示（delivery）方面，演讲者虽带有口音，但语速适中，语意表达清楚。而图片、文字和视频这些视觉辅助手段（visual aids）的使用也让整个演讲的内容变得更加清晰生动。

精彩加油站

This Gel Can Make You Stop Bleeding Instantly
可以立即止血的凝胶

精彩视频

I want you guys to imagine that you're a soldier running through the battlefield. Now, you're shot in the leg with a bullet, which severs your femoral artery. Now, this bleed is extremely traumatic and can kill you in less than three minutes. Unfortunately, by the time that a medic actually gets to you, what the medic has on his or her belt can take five minutes or more, with the application of pressure, to stop that type of bleed.

Now, this problem is not only a huge problem for the military, but it's also a huge problem that's epidemic throughout the entire medical field, which is how do we actually look at wounds and how do we stop them quickly in a way that can work with the body.

So now, what I've been working on for the last four years is to develop smart biomaterials, which are actually materials that will work with the body, helping it to heal and helping it to allow the wounds to heal normally.

我们来想象一下：你是一名正在战场上冲锋陷阵的战士。可是，你的腿上中了一枪，打断了股动脉。血流得很快，三分钟之内你就可能毙命。更不幸的是，如果等到医疗兵过来，用腰间设备以按压方式，起码要五分钟以上才能止血。

现在，这个问题已经不只是军队要解决的大问题，它同样也是涉及整个医学界的大问题，它涉及我们究竟该如何看待伤口，我们如何通过一种符合身体运行机制的方法尽快止血。

所以，我在过去四年里一直致力于开发智能的生物材料。这些生物材料可以很好地促进身体复原，并且帮助伤口正常愈合。

So now, before we do this, we have to take a much closer look at actually how does the body work. So now, everybody here knows that the body is made up of cells. So the cell is the most basic unit of life. But not many people know what else. But it actually turns out that your cells sit in this mesh of complicated fibers, proteins and sugars known as the extracellular matrix. So now, the ECM is actually this mesh that holds the cells in place, provides structure for your tissues, but it also gives the cells a home. It allows them to feel what they're doing, where they are, and tells them how to act and how to behave.

And it actually turns out that the extracellular matrix is different from every single part of the body. So the ECM in my skin is different than the ECM in my liver, and the ECM in different parts of the same organ actually vary, so it's very difficult to be able to have a product that will react to the local extracellular matrix, which is exactly what we're trying to do. So now, for example, think of the rainforest. You have the canopy, you have the understory, and you have the forest floor. Now, all of these parts of the forest are made up of different plants, and different animals call them home. So just like that, the extracellular matrix is incredibly diverse in three

但是在讲到这些之前,我们要仔细地研究一下身体究竟是怎么运作的。在座各位都知道,身体是由细胞构成的,细胞是构成生命的最基本单位。但是大多数人对其他的却了解不多。事实上,这些细胞散落在错综复杂的纤维、蛋白质和糖之间,它们被统称为细胞外基质。细胞外基质(ECM)其实就是一个可以固定细胞的网架结构,为组织结构提供支撑,同样也为细胞提供了容身之所。细胞外基质可以使细胞了解它们在做些什么,它们在哪里,并且告诉它们该怎样运作,怎样表现。

另外,在身体的不同部位,细胞外基质实际上是不一样的。就是说,我皮肤上的细胞外基质与我肝脏上的细胞外基质是不同的。并且在同一个器官上,细胞外基质也会有所不同。因此很难生产出这样一种产品,它可以跟不同部位的细胞外基质产生反应,而这正是我们在努力做的事情。举一个例子,想象一片热带雨林,有树冠层、灌木层和地面层。这三部分孕育着不同的植物和动物。就像雨林一样,细胞外基质在三维空间内有令人难以想象的多样性。另外,细胞外基质负责所有伤口愈合的工作。假如你划伤了身体,你需要重建这个非常复杂

dimensions. On top of that, the extracellular matrix is responsible for all wound healing, so if you imagine cutting the body, you actually have to rebuild this very complex ECM in order to get it to form again, and a scar, in fact, is actually poorly formed extracellular matrix.

So now, behind me is an animation of the extracellular matrix. So as you see, your cells sit in this complicated mesh and as you move throughout the tissue, the extracellular matrix changes. So now every other piece of technology on the market can only manage a two-dimensional approximation of the extracellular matrix, which means that it doesn't fit in with the tissue itself.

So when I was a freshman at NYU, what I discovered was you could actually take small pieces of plant-derived polymers and reassemble them onto the wound. So if you have a bleeding wound like the one behind me, you can actually put our material onto this, and just like Lego blocks, it'll reassemble into the local tissue. So that means if you put it onto liver, it turns into something that looks like liver, and if you put it onto skin, it turns into something that looks just like skin. So when you put the gel on, it actually reassembles into this local tissue. So now, this has a whole bunch of applications, but basically the idea is,

的细胞外基质，以便让这个伤口重新愈合。伤疤其实就是重新形成的细胞外基质，只是没那么美观而已。

那么现在我身后放映的，是一个细胞外基质的动画。你可以看到，细胞坐落在这个复杂的网络中，并且随着组织结构的移动，细胞外基质也在变化着。所以，现有市场上的技术只能管理二维的细胞外基质，这就意味着不能适应组织结构。

当我还是纽约大学的新生时，我发现可以提取小片植物中的聚合物，然后让它们在伤口上面重新聚合。如果你有类似动画中正在流血的伤口，你可以把我们的材料涂抹在这个伤口上面，就像是乐高砖块一样，它会与所在部位的组织重新聚合。这就意味着如果你把它涂在肝脏上，它会转化成类似肝组织的东西；如果你把它涂在皮肤上，它会变成类似皮肤组织的东西。就是说当你涂上这种凝胶，它会和相应部位的组织重新聚合。这个材料有多种用途。最基本的思想就是，不管你把这个产品涂在哪里，它都可以

wherever you put this product, you're able to reassemble into it immediately.

Now, this is a simulated arterial bleed—blood warning—at twice human artery pressure. So now, this type of bleed is incredibly traumatic, and like I said before, would actually take five minutes or more with pressure to be able to stop. Now, in the time that it takes me to introduce the bleed itself, our material is able to stop that bleed, and it's because it actually goes on and works with the body to heal, so it reassembles into this piece of meat, and then the blood actually recognizes that that's happening, and produces fibrin, producing a very fast clot in less than 10 seconds.

So now this technology, by January, will be in the hands of veterinarians, and we're working very diligently to try to get it into the hands of doctors, hopefully within the next year.

But really, once again, I want you guys to imagine that you are a soldier running through a battlefield. Now, you get hit in the leg with a bullet, and instead of bleeding out in three minutes, you pull a small pack of gel out of your belt, and with the press of a button, you're able to stop your own bleed and you're on your way to recovery.

Thank you very much.

很快地和所在部位的组织重新聚合。

这是一个模拟动脉出血的场景,出血量已经达到警戒级别,是人类动脉压的两倍。这种出血状况是很严重的。就像我之前说过的那样,要止住流血,需要至少五分钟。现在,就在我介绍这个伤口的这会,我们的材料已经止住流血了,这是因为它可以与身体作用,和这块肉聚合在一起,血流识别出这一反应,产生纤维蛋白,然后在十秒钟之内很快地凝结成伤疤。

所以到一月份的时候,兽医将会率先使用这项技术。我们希望在接下来的一年中,我们的努力可以让该技术也能为医生所用。

再一次,我希望你们可以想象下这幅画面,你是一个士兵,奔跑在战场上。现在,你腿上中了一枪,这一次,你没有让血在三分钟之内流尽。你从腰间拿出了一小盒我们的凝胶,按下按钮,你为自己止了血,而你的伤情也正在好转。

非常感谢。

Lecture 4   Welcome to the Genomic Revolution

欢迎进入基因革命时代

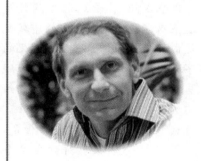

　　理查德·雷斯尼克(Richard Resnick)是 GenomeQuest（GQ）的首席执行官，这是一家专门为基因组医学研究而开发软件的生命科技公司。基因组医学研究以人类基因组为基础，将生命科学与临床医学整合在一起，通过基因组的处理进行人类医学研究，并提供更具针对性的治疗。在此之前，理查德曾是 Mosaic Bioinformatics 公司的首席执行官，曾经参加过由麻省理工学院埃里克·兰德主持的人类基因组研究项目。

1　Ladies and gentlemen, I present to you the human genome.

2　*Chromosome*① one—top left, bottom right—are the sex chromosomes. Women have two copies of that big X chromosome; men have the X and, of course, that small copy of the Y. Sorry boys, but it's just a tiny little thing that makes you different. So if you zoom in on this genome, then what you see, of course, is this double-helix structure—the code of life spelled out with these four biochemical letters, or we call them bases: A, C, G and T. How many are there in the human genome? Three billion. Is that a big number? Well, everybody can throw around big numbers. But in fact, if I were to place one base on each pixel of this 1,280 × 800-resolution screen, we would need 3,000 screens to take a look at the genome. So it's really quite big.

3　And perhaps because of its size, a group of people—all, by the way, with Y chromosomes—decided they would want to sequence it.

4　And so 15 years, actually, and about four

1　女士们、先生们,这就是人类基因组。

2　左上角是一号染色体,右下角是性染色体。女性有两条大大的X染色体,男性有一个X。当然,还有个小小的Y。不好意思了,各位男士们,让你们与众不同的只是那一个小东西。如果放大这条基因组,你看到的当然就是这个双螺旋结构。生命的密码就是由A,C,G和T这几个生化的字符组成的,我们也可称之为碱基。人类基因组有多少这样的结构呢?30亿。这个数字大吧?当然了,大数字到处都是。但是,如果我把一个碱基对放在这个1 280×800屏幕的一个像素上,得要3 000块屏幕才能一睹人类基因组的全貌。所以这个数字真的很大。

3　也许因为这个数字太大了,于是一群人——补充说明一下,是一群有着Y染色体的人——他们决定对它们进行测序。

4　在耗费了15年的光阴,烧金

---

① chromosome *n.* 染色体

billion dollars later, the genome was sequenced and published. In 2003, the final version was published, and they keep working on it. That was all done on a machine like this. It costs about a dollar for each base—a very slow way of doing it.

5   Well, folks, I'm here to tell you that the world has completely changed, and none of you know about it. So now what we do is take a genome, we make maybe 50 copies of it, we cut all those copies up into little 50-base reads, and then we sequence them, massively parallel. Then we bring that into software and reassemble it, and tell you what the story is. So to give you a picture of what this looks like, the Human Genome Project: 3 gigabases, right? One run on one of these modern machines: 200 gigabases in a week. And that 200 is going to change to 600 this summer, and there's no sign of this pace slowing. The price of a base, to sequence a base, has fallen 100 million times. That's the equivalent of you filling up your car with gas in 1998, waiting until 2011, and now you can drive to Jupiter and back twice.

40 亿美元之后,对基因组的测序终于完成并发表了。2003 年,最终的版本面世了,但完善的工作仍在继续。这些工作都是在这样一台机器上完成的。每个碱基对测序大概要花费 1 美元左右,而且排序速度非常慢。

5   不过各位,我今天来要告诉你们,这个世界已经在不知不觉中发生了翻天覆地的变化。现在我们可以把一个基因组复制 50 份,然后将它们切割为 50 个碱基序列,再进行大规模同时测序。然后我们把结果导入软件,重新组合一下,这就是你们看到的结果了。我这样来解释可能更直观一些:人类基因组计划一共有 30 亿碱基对,对吧? 在这些现代机器上进行测序的话,每周可以完成 2 000 亿碱基对。而这个夏天它的速度会提高到每周 6 000 亿,并且这个速度有可能还会提高。测序一个碱基对的费用下跌了一亿倍。这就相当于你在 1998 年给汽车加满一次油的钱,放到 2011 年可以让你在地球和木星来回开两次。

⁶ World population，PC placements，the *archive*① of all of medical literature，Moore's law，the old way of sequencing，and here's all the new stuff. Guys，this is a log scale；you don't typically see lines that go up like that. So the worldwide capacity to sequence human genomes is something like 50，000 to 100，000 human genomes this year. We know this based on the machines that are being placed. This is expected to double，triple or maybe quadruple year over year for the foreseeable future. In fact，there's one lab in particular that represents 20 percent of all that capacity. It's called the Beijing Genomics Institute. The Chinese are absolutely winning this race to the new Moon，by the way. What does this mean for medicine？

⁷ So a woman，age 37，presents with stage 2 *estrogen*② receptor-positive breast cancer. She is treated with surgery，*chemotherapy*③ and radiation. She goes home. Two years later，she comes back with stage 3 C ovarian cancer，unfortunately；treated again with surgery and chemotherapy. She comes back three years later at age 42 with more ovarian cancer，more chemotherapy. Six months later，she comes

6   世界人口、电脑普及、所有医学文献的存档、摩尔定律、早期的排序方式，而这条曲线代表着我们的新技术（图表）。各位，这可是个对数尺度，通常你是看不到这样上升的走势的。世界范围内对人类基因组测序的能力在今年可以达到五万到十万个人类基因组。我们是从已经投入应用的机器来估算的。在可预见的未来里，每年这个数字都会翻倍，或是以三倍甚至四倍的速度增长。实际上，有一个实验室占据了全世界测序能力的 20%。它就是"华大基因"。中国毫无疑问在这场新的"登月竞赛"中处于领先。那么这个技术对于医学意味着什么呢？

7   有一位女士，37 岁，被查出患有二期雌激素受体阳性乳腺癌。在经历了手术、化疗和放疗后，回到了家里。不幸的是，两年后，她又被发现患上了卵巢癌三期 C 并再次接受手术和化疗。三年后她 42 岁，因卵巢癌发展，再次回到医院，接受更多的化疗。6 个月后，她又因患上了急性骨

---

① archive *n.* 档案
② estrogen *n.* 雌性激素
③ chemotherapy *n.* 化疗

back with *acute myeloid leukemia*①. She goes into *respiratory failure*② and dies eight days later.

髓性白血病再次入院,最终因呼吸衰竭在八天后去世。

8　So first: the way in which this woman was treated, in as little as 10 years, will look like bloodletting. And it's because of it, people like my colleague, Rick Wilson, at the Genome Institute at Washington University, who decided to take a look at this woman *postmortem*③. And he took skin cells, healthy skin and cancerous *bone marrow*④, and sequenced the whole genomes of both of them in a couple of weeks, no big deal. Then he compared those two genomes in software, and what he found, among other things, was a deletion—a 2,000-base deletion across three billion bases in a particular gene called TP53. If you have this *deleterious*⑤ *mutation*⑥ in this gene, you're 90 percent likely to get cancer in your life.

8　在短短的 10 年中,这名女性接受的治疗看起来就如同放血一般。因此,我一位在华盛顿大学基因组研究所工作的同事瑞克·威尔逊决定要将这名女性的遗体进行检验。他提取了她的皮肤细胞,健康的皮肤以及癌化的骨髓,并在几周的时间内对两整套基因组进行了测序——这工作量现在根本不算事儿了。然后他通过软件比对两个基因组,并在 30 亿碱基对中一个叫做 TP53 的基因上他发现了一段 2 000 碱基对的基因缺损。如果这个基因上有此类缺损的突变,那么患上癌症的可能性高达 90%。

9　So unfortunately, this doesn't help this woman, but it does have severe—profound, if you will—implications to her family. I mean, if

9　很不幸,这个发现并没能帮上这位女士,但对她的家人却有着非常重要的意义。我的意思

---

①　acute myeloid leukemia 急性髓性白血病
②　respiratory failure 呼吸衰竭
③　postmortem *n.* 尸体解剖
④　bone marrow *n.* 骨髓
⑤　deleterious *adj.* 有害的
⑥　mutation *n.* (遗)突变

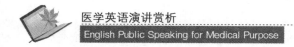

they have the same mutation, and they get this genetic test and they understand it, then they can get regular screens and can catch cancer early, and potentially live a significantly longer life.

是,如果他们存在相同的基因突变,基因检测就可以让他们了解到这一点,那样就可以通过定期筛检,及早发现癌症,并有可能显著提高他们的寿命。

10   Let me introduce you to the Beery twins, diagnosed with *cerebral palsy*① at the age of two. Their mom is a very brave woman who didn't believe it; the symptoms weren't matching up. And through some heroic efforts and a lot of Internet searching, she was able to convince the medical community that, in fact, they had something else. They had dopa-responsive *dystonia*②. And so they were given L-Dopa, and their symptoms did improve, but they weren't totally *asymptomatic*③. Significant problems remained.

10   让我来介绍一下毕瑞兄妹俩。他们在 2 岁时被诊断出脑瘫。他们的母亲是个非常勇敢的女性,她坚信脑瘫并不是真正的病因,因为实际症状与诊断并不相符。通过不懈的努力和大量的网上搜索,她成功地说服医疗人员,实际上孩子患上的是另一种病。他们所患的是多巴反应性肌张力失常。于是医生改用左旋多巴进行治疗,症状确实得到了改善,但是并没有完全消除,目前还有一些严重问题有待解决。

11   Turns out the gentleman in this picture is a guy named Joe Beery, who was lucky enough to be the CIO of a company called Life Technologies. They're one of two companies that makes these massive whole-genome sequencing tools. And so he got his kids sequenced. What they found was a series of

11   照片里的这位男士名叫乔·毕瑞,很幸运的是,他是一家名叫生命科技公司的首席信息官。这家公司是提供基因组测序设备的两大现有供应商之一。他对自己孩子的基因进行了测序。结果在一个叫做 SPR 的基因上发现一

---

① cerebral palsy 脑瘫

② dystonia *n.* 肌张力障碍

③ asymptomatic *adj.* 无症状的

mutations in a gene called SPR, which is responsible for producing *serotonin*①, among other things. So on top of L-Dopa, they gave these kids a serotonin precursor drug, and they're effectively normal now. Guys, this would never have happened without whole-genome sequencing. At the time—this was a few years ago—it cost $100,000. Today it's $10,000, next year, $1,000, the year after, $100, give or take a year. That's how fast this is moving.

12　So here's little Nick—likes Batman and squirt guns. And it turns out Nick shows up at the children's hospital with this *distended*② belly, like a famine victim. And it's not that he's not eating; it's that when he eats, his *intestine*③ basically opens up and *feces*④ spill out into his *gut*⑤. So a hundred surgeries later, he looks at his mom and says, "Mom, please pray for me. I'm in so much pain." His *pediatrician*⑥ happens to have a background in *clinical genetics*⑦ and he has no idea what's going on, but he says, "Let's get this kid's genome sequenced." And what they find is a

系列突变。这个基因负责产生的物质里包括血清素。所以在左旋多巴的基础上，他们又给两个孩子使用了血清素前体药物，现在他们已经完全正常了。各位，如果没有全基因组测序，这些是永远不可能实现的。几年前，全基因测序的花费高达十万美元，而如今的价格却只有一万，明年有可能是一千，到了后年或者大后年就会是一百了。价格的变动就是如此之快。

12　这是小尼克，喜欢蝙蝠侠和水枪。尼克来到儿童医院时，他的肚子肿胀得像是正经历饥荒的小孩。他并不是没有吃东西，而是无论他吃什么，肠道都会自动打开，排泄物溢出到他的腹腔内。经历了无数次的手术后，他看着妈妈说："妈妈，为我祷告吧，我真是太疼了。"他的儿科医生恰好有临床遗传学方面的背景，他虽然不知道病因到底是什么，但他还是说："我们给这个孩子做个基因测序吧。"他发现在一个控制程序

---

① serotonin *n.* 血清素
② distended *adj.* 膨胀的，扩张的
③ intestine *n.* 肠
④ feces *n.* 排泄物，粪便
⑤ gut *n.* 内脏
⑥ pediatrician *n.* 儿科医生
⑦ clinical genetics *n.* 临床遗传学

single-point mutation in a gene responsible for controlling programmed cell death. So the theory is that he's having some immunological reaction to what's going on—to the food, essentially. And that's a natural reaction, which causes some programmed cell death, but the gene that regulates that down is broken. And so this informs, among other things, of course, a treatment for bone marrow transplant, which he undertakes. And after nine months of grueling recovery, he's now eating steak with A1 sauce.

13   The prospect of using the genome as a universal diagnostic is upon us today. Today. It's here. And what it means for all of us is that everybody in this room could live an extra 5, 10, 20 years, just because of this one thing. Which is a fantastic story, unless you think about humanity's footprint on the planet, and our ability to keep up food production. So it turns out that the very same technology is also being used to grow new lines of corn, wheat, soybean and other crops that are highly tolerant of drought, of flood, of pests and pesticides. Now, look—as long as we continue to increase the population, we'll have to continue to grow and eat genetically modified foods. And that's the only position I'll take today. Unless there's anybody in the audience who'd like to volunteer to stop eating. None, not one.

性细胞死亡的基因上有一处单点突变。所以问题就出在他的身体对吃下去的食物产生了一种免疫反应。这原本是很正常的一种反应,它会导致程序性细胞死亡,但是负责抑制这个机制的基因失效了。了解了这些以后,医生们当然就知道该怎么做了,他们在他的治疗方案中加入了骨髓移植。在经历了9个月痛苦的恢复期后,他现在可以沾着A1酱汁吃牛排了。

13　如今,使用基因组来作为常规诊断方法就快要成为现实。它现在已经触手可及。对于我们所有人而言,这项技术意味着,在座的各位可以多活五年、十年或者是二十年。这真是太棒了,当然前提是你不去考虑人类对地球的破坏以及食物产量能否跟得上的问题。可其实同样的技术也是能用来培育具有更强的抗旱力、抗涝力、抗虫性和抗药性的新型玉米、麦子、大豆和其他作物的。现在,你们都明白了吧——只要人口继续增长,我们就必须种植和食用转基因食物。这是我今天唯一要声明的立场。当然除非我们观众里有人想绝食的。没有人,谁都不想。

14　This is a typewriter, a staple of every desktop for decades. And, in fact, the typewriter was essentially deleted by this thing. And then more general versions of word processors came about. But ultimately, it was a disruption on top of a disruption. It was Bob Metcalfe inventing the Ethernet, and the connection of all these computers that fundamentally changed everything. Suddenly we had Netscape, we had Yahoo. And we had, indeed, the entire dot-com bubble. Not to worry though, that was quickly rescued by the iPod, Facebook and, indeed, Angry Birds.

15　Look, this is where we are today. This is the genomic revolution today. This is where we are. What I'd like you to consider is: What does it mean when these dots don't represent the individual bases of your genome, but they connect to genomes all across the planet? I just recently had to buy life insurance, and I was required to answer: A. I have never had a genetic test; B. I've had one, here you go; or C. I've had one and I'm not telling. Thankfully, I was able to answer A, and I say that honestly, in case my life insurance agent is listening. But what would have happened if I had said C?

14　这是个打字机,几十年的时间里,它一直是所有办公桌上的必备用品。接着,打字机几乎被这台设备淘汰了。然后一代又一代的文字处理机出现了。但最终,长江后浪推前浪,更加颠覆性的技术来了。鲍勃·梅得卡夫发明了以太网,连接起了所有电脑,彻底地改变了一切。突然间我们有了网景,有了雅虎,再然后我们有了整个互联网的泡沫经济。不过别担心,iPod,脸书很快就拯救了我们,当然,还有愤怒的小鸟。

15　看到了吧,这就是我们现在的状况。这就是如今的基因革命。我希望你们思考的是:当这些小点代表的不再是你个人基因里的碱基,而是把它们与全世界的基因联系在一起,这会意味着什么? 我最近刚买了人身保险。我被要求在下面选项中作出选择:A. 我从没有做过基因测试;B. 我做过基因测试(那你就没戏了);和 C. 我做过基因测试,但我不告诉你。还好我可以选 A。我的保险经纪人有可能也会听到这个演讲,所以我必须申明我的回答是诚实的。可如果我选了C,那又会是什么结果呢?

16　Consumer applications for genomics will flourish. Do you want to see if you're genetically compatible with your girlfriend? Sure. DNA sequencing on your iPhone? There's an app for that. Personalized genomic massage, anyone? There's already a lab today that tests for *allele*① 334 of the AVPR1 gene, the so-called cheating gene. So anybody who's here today with your significant other, just turn over to them, *swab*② their mouth, send it to the lab and you'll know for sure. Do you really want to elect a president whose genome suggests *cardiomyopathy*③? Think of it—it's 2016, and the leading candidate releases not only her four years of back-tax returns, but also her personal genome. And it looks really good. Then she challenges all her competitors to do the same. Do you think that's not going to happen? Do you think it would have helped John McCain?

16　与基因组相关的消费者应用软件会遍地开花。你想了解自己跟女友基因上是否适合？当然可以。想在你的 iPhone 上做 DNA 测序？也有这么个应用。个性化的基因按摩，有人想试试吗？现在已经有实验室可以测试 AVPR1 基因上的等位基因 334 了，也就是所谓的出轨基因。所以现场如果有谁带了你的另一半来，也想知道他（她）是否忠贞的话，只要转向他（她），用棉签在他（她）嘴里刮一下，送到实验室去，你就会知道结果了。你会选举一位基因显示有心肌病隐患的总统吗？设想一下这样的情景，2016 年的时候，领先的总统竞选人不仅公布了她过去四年的税务清单，也公开了她的个人基因组。听上去很不错吧。然后这位竞选者也要求她的竞争对手做同样的事情。你不认为这会发生吗？你觉得这会不会帮到约翰·麦凯恩？

17　How many people in the audience have the last name Resnick, like me? Raise your hand. Anybody? Nobody. Typically, there's one or

17　观众里有多少人跟我一样是姓雷斯尼克的？请举手。有吗？没有。通常会有一两个。我父亲

---

① allele *n.* 等位基因
② swab *v.* 擦拭，涂抹（药）于
③ cardiomyopathy *n.* 心肌症

two. So my father's father was one of 10 Resnick brothers. They all hated each other, and all moved to different parts of the planet. So it's likely I'm related to every Resnick that I ever meet, but I don't know. So imagine if my genome were de-identified, sitting in software, and a third cousin's genome was also sitting there, and there was software that could compare the two and make these associations. Not hard to imagine. My company has software that does this right now. Imagine one more thing, that that software is able to ask both parties for mutual *consent*①: "Would you be willing to meet your third cousin?" And if we both say yes—voilà! Welcome to Chromosomally LinkedIn.

18　Now this is probably a good thing, right? Bigger clan gatherings and so on. But maybe it's a bad thing as well. How many fathers in the room? Raise your hands. OK, so experts think that one to three percent of you are not actually the father of your child.

19　Look—These genomes, these 23 chromosomes, they don't in any way represent the quality of our relationships or the nature of our society—at least not yet. And like any new

的父亲是 10 个雷斯尼克兄弟中的一个。他们都互相讨厌，就搬到了世界各地生活。所以有可能我与我遇到过的每一个雷斯尼克都有亲戚关系，只是我不知道而已。试想如果我的基因被辨识，并记录在了软件里，然后我的一个远房表兄的基因也被记录了下来，有软件可以比较这两组基因，并作出关联。这一切并不难想象。我的公司现在就有这样的软件。再想象一下，这个软件还可以征求双方的同意："你想不想与你的远房表兄见面？"如果两人都同意了——哇啦！欢迎登录染色体领英网。

18　现在看来这也许是个好事，对吧？能集合更多的家族成员或者其他什么的。但也可能是坏事。这屋子里有多少做父亲的请举手。好吧，专家认为你们中间有 1% 到 3% 的人并不是你孩子的父亲。

19　请看——这些基因组，这 23 对染色体。它们并不能反映人与人之间的关系，或是我们这个社会的本质——至少目前还不能。

---

① consent *n.* 同意

technology, it's really in humanity's hands to wield it for the betterment of mankind or not. And so I urge you all to wake up and to tune in and to influence the genomic revolution that's happening all around you.

如同任何新科技一样，它的好坏完全取决于人类是否将它使用在对人类有益处的地方。所以我热切地期望大家都能领悟，都能关注，并且参与到这场发生在你们身边的基因革命里来。

20 Thank you.

20 谢谢。

 演讲赏析

这篇演讲的前半部分属于说解性演讲（informative speech），演讲者对于人类基因组的测序做了解说和展示，内容包括基因测序的起源、实验方法、技术发展以及在人类疾病治疗过程中的使用和实际效果。演讲者从自己从事的领域出发，深入探讨了一个自己所熟知、了解的话题（topic），而话题本身也显示了研究和讨论的价值，以及对听众的吸引力，因此，该演讲从话题选择的角度而言，已经具备了一篇成功演讲的条件和可能。

演讲主体部分主要按照话题顺序（topical order）进行组织，包括基因测序用于医学研究和临床治疗的发展过程，三个案例的展示分析，基因测序在其他领域内的应用及未来发展前景等。有序的内容安排，可以提高演讲的表现力，也利于听众的理解。

演讲者在观点展开及论述方面，充分利用了例证（examples）和数据（statistics）的表现效果。他引用多个延展例证（extended examples），对比使用基因测序诊断疾病前后、在治疗方案和治疗效果上的差异，来说明基因测序的方法在医学实践中的意义和价值。基因测序不仅可以发现基因突变、帮助预见癌变，也能够为某些临床症状找到真正的病因。同时，演讲者还使用了雷斯尼克兄弟的假想例证（hypothetical example）。这些例证要么引发了听众对病人的同情，要么吸引了听众对主题——基因测序作用的关注，保证了演讲过程中以听众为中心（audience-centered）。此外，演讲者对数据的使用和解释也给我们留下了深刻的印象,例如第一段里对碱基对数量这一天文数字的形象解释,还有第四段中基因测序费用的降幅描述,都是生动解释枯燥数字的极好范例。

演讲中大量形式多样的视觉辅助(visual aids)的使用,也是本篇演讲的一大特色。这些视觉辅助包括图片(photographs)、线状图表(line graph)、柱状图表(bar graph)等。在展示图片、图表的同时,演讲者做了相应的解释和说明(explain visual aids),因而可以更加充分地发挥视觉辅助的作用。

演讲的后半部分属于说服类演讲(a persuasive speech),话题也由基因测序在医学中的实践转向其他领域内的拓展和应用,包括备受争议的转基因食品的种植和食用。演讲的最后部分呼吁观众对基因革命的影响做深刻的思考,基因革命和我们的生活密切相关,会影响甚至改变我们的生活方式。

演讲者的语速稍快,但演讲过程中比较放松,演讲内容风趣幽默,能够很好地与观众互动,并时常得到观众的反馈。

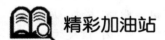 精彩加油站

Your Genes Are Not Your Fate
基因决定不了你的命运

精彩视频

One way to change our genes is to make new ones, as Craig Venter has so elegantly shown. Another is to change our lifestyles. And what we're learning is how powerful and dynamic these changes can be, that you don't have to wait very long to see the benefits. When you eat healthier, manage stress, exercise and love more, your brain actually gets more blood flow and more oxygen. But more than that, your brain gets measurably

改变基因的一个方法是制造出新的基因,正如克雷格·文特尔给我们完美地展示过的那样。另一个方法则是改变我们的生活习惯。而我们发现,后者带来的变化是如此强大,我们无须等待很长时间就能看到成效。当你吃得更加健康、懂得管理压力、坚持锻炼身体并且付出爱心的时候,你的大脑实际上会获得更多的供血与供氧。而且你的

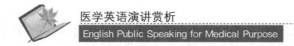
bigger. Things that were thought impossible just a few years ago can actually be measured now. This was figured out by Robin Williams a few years before the rest of us.

Now, there's something you can do to make your brain grow new brain cells. Some of my favorite things, like chocolate and tea, blueberries, alcohol in moderation, stress management and cannabinoids found in marijuana. I'm just the messenger. (Laughter) What were we just talking about? (Laughter) And other things that can make it worse, that can cause you to lose brain cells. The usual suspects, like saturated fat and sugar, nicotine, opiates, cocaine, too much alcohol and chronic stress.

Your skin gets more blood flow when you change your lifestyle, so you age less quickly. Your skin doesn't wrinkle as much. Your heart gets more blood flow. We've shown that you can actually reverse heart disease. That these clogged arteries that you see on the upper left, after only a year become measurably less clogged. And the cardiac PET scan shown on the lower left, the blue means no blood flow. A year later—orange and white is maximum blood flow. We've shown you may be able to stop and reverse the progression of early prostate

大脑在体积上也会有所增长。几年前，我们还以为这种增长是无法测量的，但现在可以了。这都要归功于罗宾·威廉姆斯，他走在了我们其他人的前面，几年前就找到了测量方法。

事实上，很多事情都可以促进新脑细胞的产生。我个人比较喜欢的有吃巧克力、喝茶、食用蓝莓、适量饮酒、调节压力及服用大麻类物质。当然啦，我只是这么说说而已（意为并无鼓励人们使用大麻的意图）。（笑声）啊，我们刚说到哪啦？（笑声）而有些东西只会适得其反，使你的脑细胞数量减少。常见的罪魁祸首有饱和脂肪、糖类、尼古丁、鸦片类物质、可卡因、过度饮酒以及慢性压力。

当你的生活习惯更为健康，皮肤的供血会更加充足，这会延缓衰老，你的皮肤就不会有那么多皱纹了。你的心脏供血也会增加。我们的研究表明，这甚至可以阻止心脏病的发作。大家可以看一下幻灯片的左上角，这里展示的是阻塞了的动脉，而仅仅一年之后，动脉的阻塞程度明显降低。我们再来看下左下角心脏的断层显像，蓝色部分表示没有血液流通。同样也是一年之后，我们看到了大块的橙色与白色，它们表示最大的血流量。我们的研

cancer and, by extension, breast cancer, simply by making these changes. We've found that tumor growth in vitro was inhibited 70 percent in the group that made these changes, whereas only nine percent in the comparison group.

These differences were highly significant. Even your sexual organs get more blood flow, so you increase sexual potency. One of the most effective anti-smoking ads was done by the Department of Health Services, showing that nicotine, which constricts your arteries, can cause a heart attack or a stroke, but it also causes impotence. Half of guys who smoke are impotent. How sexy is that?

Now we're also about to publish a study—the first study showing you can change gene expression in men with prostate cancer. This is what's called a heat map—and the different colors—and along the side, on the right, are different genes. And we found that over 500 genes were favorably changed—in effect, turning on the good genes, the disease-preventing genes, turning off the disease-promoting genes.

And so these findings I think are really very powerful, giving many people new hope and new choices. And companies like Navigenics and DNA Direct and 23andMe,

究还表明,仅仅通过改变不良的生活习惯,你可以阻止甚至逆转早期的前列腺癌,乃至乳腺癌。通过肿瘤生长的体外试管实验,我们发现,实验组中的肿瘤生长被抑制了70%,而在对照组中这个比例却只有9%。

这些对比是非常显著的。你的性器官也会有更多的血液供给,从而提高性能力。在所有最有效的禁烟广告中,有一则是卫生署拍摄的。这则广告说尼古丁不仅会紧缩动脉、导致心脏病或中风,它还会导致性无能。男性吸烟者中有一半是性无能者,这听起来不那么性感了吧?

最近我们还准备发表一项调查研究——首个显示罹患前列腺癌的男性有能力改变他们的基因表达的研究。这张幻灯片就是我们所说的"热图",它用不同的颜色代表不同的属性。右图显示的是变化了的基因。我们发现有500多个基因发生了良性变异,换句话说,就是那些好的、能够预防疾病的基因被激活了,而那些会引发疾病的基因被关闭了。

我认为这些发现影响巨大,能给很多人带来新的希望和选择。那些为客户提供个人基因档案的公司,比如"基因导航"、"DNA直通

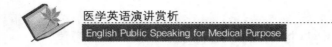
that are giving you your genetic profiles, are giving some people a sense of, "Gosh, well, what can I do about it?" Well, our genes are not our fate, and if we make these changes— they're a predisposition—but if we make bigger changes than we might have made otherwise, we can actually change how our genes are expressed. Thank you. (Applause)

车"和"染色体与我",常给客户造成这样一种感觉:"天哪,我该怎么办呢?"幸好我们的基因并不是不可改变的。即使我们有易染病体质,但如果我们做出积极的改变,做出超乎寻常的积极改变,我们真的可以改变我们的基因表达。谢谢。(鼓掌)

Lecture 5   Zombie Roaches and Other Parasite Tales

寄生虫的逆袭

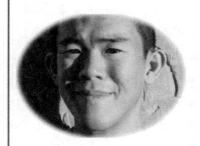

　　艾德·杨(Ed Yong)是一名英国科学记者,他的科普写作被描述为"未来科技新闻",他也因为自己的工作获得了无数的奖项。他的描写对象主要是人类以外的生命,无论是黑猩猩还是史前朱鹮,或是吸血蜘蛛,他都感兴趣。一些其貌不扬的动植物,在研究者的眼里浑身是宝,它们的生活习性和群体特征都可能会给研究者带来不小的发现,而艾德·杨以广博的搜集发现了这些研究,透过这些研究者的慧眼,了解了隐藏在幕后的鲜为人知的动植物特性,并通过他的文字把这些有趣的信息生动地传递到了读者面前。在 TED 的一次演讲中,艾德·杨解释了寄生虫是如何在自然界利用其神秘的武器和高超的本领,不知不觉而又轻而易举地操控着各种动物的行为,从而达到其隐藏的目的。难道寄生虫也在操控我们人类? 真的很有可能哟! 请听听这个新奇、幽默并有点令人毛骨悚然的演讲。

1   A herd of wildebeests, a shoal of fish, a flock of birds. Many animals gather in large groups that are among the most wonderful spectacles in the natural world. But why do these groups form? The common answers include things like seeking safety in numbers or hunting in packs or gathering to mate or breed, and all of these explanations, while often true, make a huge assumption about animal behavior, that the animals are in control of their own actions, that they are in charge of their bodies. And that is often not the case.

2   This is Artemia, a brine shrimp. You probably know it better as a sea monkey. It's small, and it typically lives alone, but it can gather in these large red swarms that span for meters, and these form because of a parasite. These shrimp are infected with a *tapeworm*①. A tapeworm is effectively a long, living gut with *genitals*② at one end and a hooked mouth at the other. As a freelance journalist, I sympathize. The tapeworm drains *nutrients*③ from Artemia's body, but it also does other things. It castrates them, it changes their color from transparent to bright red, it makes them live longer, and as biologist Nicolas Rode has found, it makes them swim in groups. Why?

1   一群角马,一群鱼,一群鸟。许多动物群居生活在一起,这是大自然中最令人惊叹的奇观之一。但是为什么这些群体会形成呢?通常的说法包括为了获得安全感、方便捕猎或者聚集以交配繁殖,所有这些解释,虽然通常是正确的,但都是建立在对动物行为的一个重要假设的基础上,那就是动物是在掌控它们自己的行为和身体。而事实往往并非如此。

2   这是卤虫,一种盐水虾。你们也许更习惯称它为海猴子。它个头很小,典型的独居类型,但是它们可以聚集成这种范围可达数米的红色群落,而原因竟是一种寄生虫。这些虾都感染了绦虫。绦虫实际上是一条长长的活着的肠子,一端是生殖器,另一端是钩状的嘴。作为一个自由撰稿人,我对它深表同情。绦虫从卤虫的体内摄取养分,但它也做其他事情。它使卤虫丧失力量,将卤虫从透明变为亮红色,延长卤虫的寿命,还有就像生物学家尼古拉斯·罗德所发现的那样,让卤虫

---

①   tapeworm *n.* 绦虫

②   genital *n.* 生殖器

③   nutrient *n.* 营养物质

Because the tapeworm, like many other *parasites*①, has a complicated life cycle involving many different *hosts*②. The shrimp are just one step on its journey. Its ultimate destination is this, the greater flamingo. Only in a flamingo can the tapeworm *reproduce*③, so to get there, it *manipulates*④ its shrimp hosts into forming these conspicuous colored swarms that are easier for a flamingo to spot and to devour, and that is the secret of the Artemia swarm. They aren't sociable through their own volition, but because they are being controlled. It's not safety in numbers. It's actually the exact opposite. The tapeworm hijacks their brains and their bodies, turning them into vehicles for getting itself into a flamingo.

成群出没。为什么呢？因为和其他许多寄生虫一样，绦虫有着复杂的生命周期，涉及许多不同的寄主。这些虾只是它旅程中的一步而已。它最终的目标是这些体型更大的火烈鸟。绦虫只有在火烈鸟体内才可以繁殖，所以为了到达那里，它操纵虾寄主们形成这些醒目的有色群落，让火烈鸟更容易去发现并吞食。这就是卤虫群的秘密。它们不是因为自身意志而聚集起来的，而是因为被控制了。它们不是通过数量优势去获得安全感。事实恰恰相反。它们的身体和大脑被绦虫劫持，变成对方的交通工具以便于让绦虫进入到一只火烈鸟的体内。

3   And here is another example of a parasitic manipulation. This is a suicidal cricket. This cricket swallowed the larvae of a Gordian worm, or horsehair worm. The worm grew to adult size within it, but it needs to get into water in order to mate, and it does that by releasing proteins that *addle*⑤ the cricket's brain, causing it to behave erratically. When

3   这里还有一个关于寄生操控的例子。这是一只自杀蟋蟀。它吞下了铁线虫（也叫马鬃虫）的幼虫。幼虫在蟋蟀体内长大成熟，但它需要到水中才能进行交配，为了完成繁殖，它通过释放一种扰乱蟋蟀大脑的蛋白质，使其行为异常。当蟋蟀靠近水体时，比如这个游泳池，它就会跳进水里

---

① parasite *n.* 寄生虫
② host *n.* 寄主
③ reproduce *v.* 繁殖
④ manipulation *n.* 操纵；控制
⑤ addle *v.* 使混乱

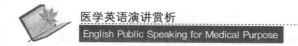
the cricket nears a body of water, such as this swimming pool, it jumps in and drowns, and the worm wriggles out of its suicidal *corpse*①. Crickets are really roomy. Who knew?

淹死，然后虫子从它的尸体中挣脱出来。蟋蟀真的是胸怀宽广啊。谁知道呢？

4   The tapeworm and the Gordian worm are not alone. They are part of an entire cavalcade of mind-controlling parasites, of fungi, viruses, and worms and insects and more that all specialize in subverting and overriding the wills of their hosts. Now, I first learned about this way of life through David Attenborough's "Trials of Life" about 20 years ago, and then later through a wonderful book called *Parasite Rex* by my friend Carl Zimmer. And I've been writing about these creatures ever since. Few topics in biology enthrall me more. It's like the parasites have subverted my own brain. Because after all, they are always compelling and they are delightfully macabre. When you write about parasites, your lexicon swells with phrases like "devoured alive" and "bursts out of its body."

4   绦虫和铁线虫并不孤单。它们是一系列专于控制思想的寄生虫、真菌、病毒、蠕虫和昆虫的一部分。我是通过大卫·阿滕伯勒大约二十年前拍的一部纪录片《生命的考验》首次了解到这种生存方式，之后又通过我的朋友卡尔·齐默尔写的一本精彩的书《寄生虫雷克斯》，对其有了进一步了解。从那时起我就一直在写这些生物。在生物学领域，很少有什么别的话题能让我更加着迷了。我的大脑就像已经被寄生虫破坏了。毕竟它们总是那么的魅力无限，在叫人毛骨悚然的同时却也能让你乐在其中。当你描写寄生虫时，你的用词里会充满了像"活活吞吃"、"冲破身体钻出来"等等这样的短语。

5   But there's more to it than that. I'm a writer, and fellow writers in the audience will know that we love stories. Parasites invite us to resist the allure of obvious stories. Their world

5   但寄生虫的魅力绝不止于此。我是一个作家，观众席中的同行们都知道，我们热爱故事。寄生虫能教我们学会抛弃那些显

---

① corpse *n.* 尸体

is one of plot twists and unexpected explanations. Why, for example, does this caterpillar start violently thrashing about when another insect gets close to it and those white cocoons that it seems to be standing guard over? Is it maybe protecting its siblings? No. This caterpillar was attacked by a parasitic wasp which laid eggs inside it. The eggs hatched and the young wasps devoured the caterpillar alive before bursting out of its body. See what I mean? Now, the caterpillar didn't die. Some of the wasps seemed to stay behind and controlled it into defending their siblings which are *metamorphosing*① into adults within those cocoons. This caterpillar is a head-banging zombie bodyguard defending the offspring of the creature that killed it.

6　We have a lot to get through. I only have 13 minutes.

7　Now, some of you are probably just desperately clawing for some solace in the idea that these things are oddities of the natural world, that they are outliers, and that point of view is understandable, because by their nature, parasites are quite small and they spend a lot of their time inside the bodies of other

而易见的故事版本。它们的世界有着太多的剧情反转和意外真相。举个例子,看这只毛毛虫,为什么当另外一只昆虫靠近它和那些白色的茧时,它就开始剧烈地颤动,就像是为了保卫那些茧一样? 难道它在保护兄弟姐妹吗? 不对。这只毛毛虫受到了一只在其体内产卵的寄生蜂的攻击。卵孵化后,幼蜂们将毛毛虫活活吞吃,再冲破其身体钻出来。现在知道我(之前)什么意思了吧? 但是,毛毛虫并没有死。有些马蜂们留了下来,并继续控制毛毛虫去保护其他茧内正在变态为成虫的马蜂兄弟姐妹们。这只毛毛虫就是一个甩头僵尸保镖,保护着杀死自己的生物的后代。

6　我们还有很多要说。但我只有 13 分钟。

7　现在,你们中有些人可能正在拼命寻找一些自我安慰的想法,认为我说的这些只是自然界中的怪异事物和个别现象,这是可以理解的,因为从本质上说,寄生虫体型微小、并且很大一部分时间生活在其他动物的体内。它

---

① metamorphose *v.* 彻底转变

things. They're easy to overlook, but that doesn't mean that they aren't important. A few years back, a man called Kevin Lafferty took a group of scientists into three Californian estuaries and they pretty much weighed and *dissected*① and recorded everything they could find, and what they found were parasites in extreme abundance. Especially common were trematodes, tiny worms that specialize in castrating their hosts like this unfortunate snail. Now, a single trematode is tiny, microscopic, but collectively they weighed as much as all the fish in the estuaries and three to nine times more than all the birds. And remember the Gordian worm that I showed you, the cricket thing? One Japanese scientist called Takuya Sato found that in one stream, these things drive so many crickets and grasshoppers into the water that the drowned insects make up some 60 percent of the diet of local trout. Manipulation is not an oddity. It is a critical and common part of the world around us, and scientists have now found hundreds of examples of such manipulators, and more excitingly, they're starting to understand exactly how these creatures control their hosts.

们容易被忽略,但这并不意味着它们不重要。几年前,一个叫凯文·拉弗蒂的人带领一组科学家前往加州的三个河口。他们几乎将所有发现的东西都仔细地进行称重、解剖和记录,最后发现寄生虫的数量极为巨大。最常见的是吸虫,它们是小小的蠕虫,专门破坏它们的寄主,就像这只不幸的蜗牛。单单一条吸虫是很小的,用显微镜才能看见,但是它们总的重量和河口所有鱼的重量相等,比河口所有鸟的重量还多三至九倍。还记得我之前向你们展示的铁线虫和那只蟋蟀么?一位名叫佐藤拓也的日本科学家在一条溪流中发现,这些虫子会把很多蟋蟀和蚱蜢带到这里,这些淹死的昆虫为当地的鲑鱼提供了百分之六十的食物。操纵已经不是一种奇特的现象了。它是我们周围世界的一个关键和普遍的组成部分,科学家们现在已经发现了数百个这样的操纵者的例子,而更令人兴奋的是,他们开始明确了解这些生物是如何控制它们的寄主的。

8　And this is one of my favorite examples. This is Ampulex compressa, the emerald

8　这是我最喜欢的例子之一。这是一只扁头泥蜂,又叫翡翠蟑

---

① dissect *v.* 进行解剖

cockroach wasp, and it is a truth universally acknowledged that an emerald cockroach wasp in possession of some *fertilized eggs*① must be in want of a cockroach. When she finds one, she stabs it with a stinger that is also a sense organ. This discovery came out three weeks ago. She stabs it with a stinger that is a sense organ equipped with small sensory bumps that allow her to feel the distinctive texture of a roach's brain. So like a person blindly rooting about in a bag, she finds the brain, and she injects it with venom into two very specific clusters of *neurons*②. Israeli scientists Frederic Libersat and Ram Gal found that the venom is a very specific chemical weapon. It doesn't kill the roach, nor does it sedate it. The roach could walk away or fly or run if it chose to, but it doesn't choose to, because the venom nixes its motivation to walk, and only that. The wasp basically un-checks the escape-from-danger box in the roach's operating system, allowing her to lead her helpless victim back to her lair by its antennae like a person walking a dog. And once there, she lays an egg on it, egg hatches, devoured alive, bursts out of body, yadda yadda yadda, you know the drill.

螳蜂，大家都知道怀有受精卵的蟑螂蜂需要蟑螂。当它找到一只蟑螂后，会用刺蛰蟑螂，那根刺实际上还是一个感觉器官。这是科学家三周前才发现的。刺上面有一些小突起，有感觉作用，蟑螂蜂就用这个具备感官功能的刺蛰蟑螂，以便于感觉到蟑螂大脑的独特质地。像一个人在袋子里瞎摸一样，蟑螂蜂最终通过这种方式找到了蟑螂的大脑，并将毒液注射到两簇特定的神经元中。以色列科学家弗雷德里克·拉波塞特和莱姆·加尔发现这个毒液是一种非常特别的化学武器。它不会杀死蟑螂，也不能将它麻醉。蟑螂如果想的话可以选择爬走、飞走或跑掉，但是它没有，因为那个毒液使其丧失了走的意愿，仅此而已。蟑螂蜂基本上关闭了蟑螂神经系统中逃避危险的本能，让其能够借助蟑螂的触角领着这位无助的受害者回到巢穴，就像人类遛狗一样。一旦到了巢穴，蟑螂蜂就在蟑螂体内产卵，卵孵化后，幼虫将蟑螂活生生吞吃，并冲破它的身体钻出来，叭啦叭啦叭啦，你们都知道是怎样一个操作了。

---

① fertilized egg 受精卵，孕卵
② neuron n. 神经元

9　Now I would argue that, once stung, the cockroach isn't a roach anymore. It's more of an extension of the wasp, just like the cricket was an extension of the Gordian worm. These hosts won't get to survive or reproduce. They have as much control over their own fates as my car. Once the parasites get in, the hosts don't get a say.

10　Now humans, of course, are no stranger to manipulation. We take drugs to shift the chemistries of our brains and to change our moods, and what are arguments or advertising or big ideas if not an attempt to influence someone else's mind? But our attempts at doing this are crude and blundering compared to the fine-grained specificity of the parasites. Don Draper only wishes he was as elegant and precise as the emerald cockroach wasp. Now, I think this is part of what makes parasites so sinister and so compelling. We place such a premium on our free will and our independence that the prospect of losing those qualities to forces unseen informs many of our deepest societal fears. Orwellian dystopias and shadowy cabals and mind-controlling supervillains—these are tropes that fill our darkest fiction, but in nature, they happen all the time.

9　现在我想说的是,蟑螂一旦被蜇了,它就不再是蟑螂了。它更像是蟑螂蜂的一个附属品,就像蟋蟀是铁线虫的附属品一样。这些寄主们无法生存和繁殖。它们对自己的命运毫无掌控力,就像我的车任由我摆布一样。一旦寄生虫进入其体内,寄主就失去了发言权。

10　当然,现在人类对于操控并不陌生。我们通过服用药物来改变我们大脑的化学反应,改变我们的情绪。还有那些辩论、广告或是伟大的想法,不都是改变他人思想的企图吗?但我们所做的与寄生虫的精确性和专业性一比,就显得粗糙和笨拙了。唐·德雷伯就希望他能像翡翠蟑螂蜂一样优雅而精确。我认为这就是寄生虫显得如此邪恶却又令人着迷的一部分原因。我们如此看重自由意志和独立自主,以至于每当意识到某种无形的力量可能会夺走这些时,便会引起深深的社会恐慌。奥威尔式的反乌托邦、见不得光的阴谋组织和善于精神控制的大反派——这些都是充斥在暗黑小说中的套路,但是在自然界中,它们无时无刻不在发生。

11   Which leads me to an obvious and disquieting question: Are there dark, sinister parasites that are influencing our behavior without us knowing about it, besides the NSA? If there are any—I've got a red dot on my forehead now, don't I? If there are any, this is a good candidate for them. This is Toxoplasma gondii, or *Toxo*①, for short, because the terrifying creature always deserves a cute nickname. Toxo infects *mammals*②, a wide variety of mammals, but it can only sexually reproduce in a cat. And scientists like Joanne Webster have shown that if Toxo gets into a rat or a mouse, it turns the *rodent* ③into a cat-seeking missile. If the infected rat smells the delightful odor of cat piss, it runs towards the source of the smell rather than the more sensible direction of away. The cat eats the rat. Toxo gets to have sex. It's a classic tale of Eat, Prey, Love. You're very charitable, generous people. Hi, Elizabeth, I loved your talk.

11   这让我想到一个显而易见且令人不安的问题:除了美国国家安全局之外,是否还有阴险邪恶的寄生虫在我们不知道的情况下操控着我们的行为? 如果有的话——是不是现在已经有人想拿把枪把我给崩了? ——如果有的话,有一个非常好的候选者。这是刚地弓形虫,简称弓虫,因为可怕的生物总得配上一个可爱点的绰号。弓虫会感染哺乳动物,各种各样的哺乳动物,但它只可以在猫体内进行有性繁殖。像乔安妮·韦伯斯特这样的科学家已经证明,如果弓虫进入老鼠体内,它就会把这只啮齿动物变成寻猫导弹。如果被感染的老鼠闻到了美妙的猫尿味道,它就会跑向气味的来源而不是明智地选择逃跑。猫吃了老鼠。弓虫去交配。这是一个关于食物、猎物、爱情的经典故事(笑点在于:这三个词的发音与一本畅销小说的书名 *Eat, Pray, Love* 相似,该书译作《美食,祈祷和恋爱》)。你们都是善良慷慨的人啊。嗨,伊丽莎白(《美食,祈祷和恋爱》的作者),我很喜欢你的演讲。

---

① Toxo *n.* 弓形虫
② mammal *n.* 哺乳动物
③ rodent *n.* 啮齿动物

12   How does the parasite control its host in this way? We don't really know. We know that Toxo releases an *enzyme*① that makes *dopamine*②, a substance involved in reward and motivation. We know it targets certain parts of a rodent's brain, including those involved in sexual arousal. But how those puzzle pieces fit together is not immediately clear. What is clear is that this thing is a single cell. This has no nervous system. It has no consciousness. It doesn't even have a body. But it's manipulating a mammal? We are mammals. We are more intelligent than a mere rat, to be sure, but our brains have the same basic structure, the same types of cells, the same chemicals running through them, and the same parasites. Estimates vary a lot, but some figures suggest that one in three people around the world have Toxo in their brains. Now typically, this doesn't lead to any overt illness. The parasite holds up in a dormant state for a long period of time. But there's some evidence that those people who are carriers score slightly differently on personality questionnaires than other people, that they have a slightly higher risk of car accidents, and there's some evidence that people with *schizophrenia*③ are more likely to be infected. Now, I think this evidence is still inconclusive, and even among

12   寄生虫到底是怎样在这种方式下操纵其寄主的？我并不真正了解。但我们知道弓虫释放一种酶,这种酶会产生一种和奖励与动机有关的物质——多巴胺。这种酶把老鼠大脑中特定的部分作为目标,包括那些涉及性冲动的部分。这些已知和未知的信息就像拼图的碎片一样,但它们究竟是怎样拼在一起的,我们现在还不是很清楚。但我们已经知道的是,弓虫是单细胞生物。它没有神经系统。它没有意识。它甚至连身体都没有。但是它却在操控一只哺乳动物？我们都是哺乳动物。毫无疑问我们比小小的老鼠更加智慧,但是我们的大脑和老鼠的大脑有着相同的基本构造、同类型的细胞、同样存在于细胞间的化学物质,以及同样的寄生虫。我们对这一切有着各不相同的猜测,但数据显示,全世界三分之一的人类大脑里都是有弓虫的。在通常情况下,它们不会导致任何显性病症。寄生虫在很长的一段时间里都会保持休眠状态。但是有一些证据显示,那些寄生虫携带者在性格调查问卷中和其他人的得分略有不同:他们

---

①   enzyme *n.* 酶
②   dopamine *n.* 多巴胺
③   schizophrenia *n.* 精神分裂症

Toxo researchers，opinion is divided as to whether the parasite is truly influencing our behavior. But given the widespread nature of such manipulations，it would be completely implausible for humans to be the only species that weren't similarly affected.

发生车祸的风险会偏高一些，还有证据显示患有精神分裂症的人更容易被弓虫感染。我认为这个证据还不是那么令人信服，而且即便在弓虫研究者内部，对于寄生虫是否能真正影响我们行为的问题也仍存在争议。但鉴于这种操控现象的普遍性，人类成为唯一没有被感染物种的可能性很低。

13　And I think that this capacity to constantly subvert our way of thinking about the world makes parasites amazing. They're constantly inviting us to look at the natural world sideways，and to ask if the behaviors we're seeing，whether they're simple and obvious or baffling and puzzling，are not the results of individuals acting through their own accord but because they are being bent to the control of something else. And while that idea may be disquieting，and while parasites' habits may be very grisly，I think that ability to surprise us makes them as wonderful and as charismatic as any panda or butterfly or dolphin.

13　我认为寄生虫这种不断颠覆我们对世界看法的能力让它们变得很神奇。它们不停地促使我们从其他角度去看待大自然，并让我们去质疑自己所见到的或简单或奇怪的行为究竟是出于个体意愿还是因为被其他东西所操控。这种想法也许令人不安，寄生虫的习性也许非常可怕，但我认为，它们这种可以让我们大跌眼镜的能力仍然使它们像熊猫、蝴蝶或海豚一样美妙和迷人。

14　At the end of *On the Origin of Species*，Charles Darwin writes about the grandeur of life，and of endless forms most beautiful and most wonderful，and I like to think he could easily have been talking about a tapeworm that

14　在《物种起源》的结尾，查尔斯·达尔文写到生命以及无限的生命形态的辉煌是最美丽、最美好的。我认为，他很有可能说的就是让虾过上群居生活的绦虫，

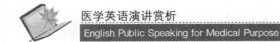
makes shrimp sociable or a wasp that takes cockroaches for walks.

或是带着蟑螂散步的黄蜂。

15　But perhaps，that's just a parasite talking.

15　但是也许，我只是被寄生虫操控在胡言乱语罢了。

16　Thank you．

16　谢谢。

 演讲赏析

　　　这是一篇说解性演讲（informative speech），一个新奇好玩、同时又令人不安的演讲。

　　　演讲者本人是一个科普作家，对自然界的奇特现象颇有研究，他选择的演讲话题（topic）"寄生虫"本身就很另类，很容易引起听众的好奇心。再看他的题目（title）——"Zombie Roaches and Other Parasite Tales"，僵尸、蟑螂、寄生虫，这个恶心的组合就够夺人眼球了，你忍不住就想知道到底发生了什么。可以说，有了一个新奇的话题和有趣的标题，演讲就成功一半了。

　　　接下来的开篇语（introduction）部分，演讲者先描绘了自然界中常见的群居现象，然后提出问题、给出常见答案，再给予否决。他并没有明确地告知大家他今天要讲的主要内容和目的，而是留下悬念，吊起听众的胃口（arouse the curiosity of the audience），是一个富有创意的开篇语设计。

　　　在主体内容（body）部分，演讲者开始举例子（examples），通过各种例子来说明寄生操控这种隐秘的自然现象的普遍存在，每个例子就是一个要点（main point），慢慢推进，不管是昆虫还是人类都和寄生虫有着联系。演讲者作为科普作家，特别擅长讲故事，加上PPT等视觉辅助工具（visual aids）的合理运用，原本深奥复杂的生物学现象被他讲得非常生动，甚至原来有些恶心的画面也变得非常有趣。在举例子的时候，演讲者也引用了专家的实验数据、结论等作为辅助材料（supporting materials），来证明这类现象的真实存在。

在结尾部分(conclusion)，演讲者指出寄生操控的存在对于人类认识大自然方式的影响，并引用(end with a quotation)达尔文在《物种起源》中的观点来概括自然界各种生命形式的神奇：*At the end of "On the Origin of Species," Charles Darwin writes about the grandeur of life, and of endless forms most beautiful and most wonderful ...*，同时也对演讲开头做了呼应(refer to the introduction)：*Many animals gather in large groups that are among the most wonderful spectacles in the natural world.*

这个演讲的时间不算短，但是听众们一直听得饶有兴趣，不时爆发出笑声和掌声。演讲者对内容的熟悉、幽默的语言和现场的发挥都为这次成功的演讲奠定了基础。

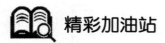 **精彩加油站**

Could We Cure HIV with Lasers?
我们能用激光治疗艾滋病吗？

精彩视频

What do you do when you have a headache? You swallow an aspirin. But for this pill to get to your head, where the pain is, it goes through your stomach, intestines and various other organs first.

Swallowing pills is the most effective and painless way of delivering any medication in the body. The downside, though, is that swallowing any medication leads to its dilution. And this is a big problem, particularly in HIV patients. When they take their anti-HIV drugs, these drugs are good

当你头痛的时候，你会怎么办？你会吞下一片阿司匹林。但在药效发挥作用之前，它要经过胃、肠和许多其他器官。

口服是最为有效，而且没有痛苦的药物输送方式。但口服会让药物稀释。这对 HIV 患者来说，是比较头疼的。当他们服用抗 HIV 药物时，会降低血液中的病毒含量，并增加 CD4 细胞（人体免疫系统中一种重要的免疫细胞）的数量。但同

for lowering the virus in the blood, and increasing the CD4 cell counts. But they are also notorious for their adverse side effects, but mostly bad, because they get diluted by the time they get to the blood, and worse, by the time they get to the sites where it matters most: within the HIV viral reservoirs. These are areas in the body—such as the lymph nodes, the nervous system, as well as the lungs—where the virus is sleeping, and will not readily get delivered in the blood of patients that are under consistent anti-HIV drugs therapy. However, upon discontinuation of therapy, the virus can awake and infect new cells in the blood.

Now, all this is a big problem in treating HIV with the current drug treatment, which is a life-long treatment that must be swallowed by patients. One day, I sat and thought, "Can we deliver anti-HIV directly within its reservoir sites, without the risk of drug dilution?" As a laser scientist, the answer was just before my eyes: Lasers, of course. If they can be used for dentistry, for diabetic wound-healing and surgery, they can be used for anything imaginable, including transporting drugs into cells.

As a matter of fact, we are currently using laser pulses to poke or drill extremely tiny holes, which open and close almost immediately in HIV-infected cells, in order

时,副作用也很大,主要是药物进入血液时已经稀释。更糟糕的是,药物到达目标位置时浓度更低,而这些地方才是关键位置,因为它们都是 HIV 病毒的储存宿主,例如淋巴结、神经系统和肺部等。在这些位置的病毒一直处于休眠中,只要病人持续服用抗 HIV 药物,病毒就不会进入病人的血液中。但是,治疗一旦中断,病毒就会苏醒并感染血液中的新细胞。

对于目前的 HIV 药物治疗,上述缺点是一个大问题,这意味着病人不得不终身服药。可有一天,我突然想到:"我们可不可以向病毒储存宿主直接注射抗 HIV 药物,这样就没有药物稀释的风险了?"作为一名激光科学家,这个问题的答案近在咫尺:当然是激光了。如果激光可以用在牙科、糖尿病的伤口愈合和外科手术上,那就可以用在任何能想到的领域,包括向细胞注射药物。

实际上,我们已经使用激光脉冲,在 HIV 感染细胞上钻出一个极小的孔。这样就可以向细胞注入药物,而且这些孔在打开后也会很快

to deliver drugs within them. "How is that possible?" you may ask. Well, we shine a very powerful but super-tiny laser beam onto the membrane of HIV-infected cells while these cells are immersed in liquid containing the drug. The laser pierces the cell, while the cell swallows the drug in a matter of microseconds. Before you even know it, the induced hole becomes immediately repaired.

Now, we are currently testing this technology in test tubes or in Petri dishes, but the goal is to get this technology in the human body, apply it in the human body. "How is that possible?" you may ask. Well, the answer is: through a three-headed device. Using the first head, which is our laser, we will make an incision in the site of infection. Using the second head, which is a camera, we meander to the site of infection. Finally, using a third head, which is a drug-spreading sprinkler, we deliver the drugs directly at the site of infection, while the laser is again used to poke those cells open.

Well, this might not seem like much right now. But one day, if successful, this technology can lead to complete eradication of HIV in the body. Yes. A cure for HIV. This is every HIV researcher's dream—in our case, a cure lead by lasers.

Thank you.

闭合。"这怎么可能?"你可能会问。是这样的,我们在把这些细胞浸泡在药物液体里的同时,将一束能量极高但极细的激光照射到细胞膜上,激光刺穿细胞,细胞瞬间就吞下了药物。在你反应过来之前,打开的孔已经修复好了。

现在,我们正在试管和培养皿中测试这项技术。我们的目标是将其应用于人类。"这怎么可能?"你可能会问。答案是一种三头的仪器。第一个探头是激光探头,用它在感染部位切一个口;第二个探头是摄像头,用来寻找感染位置;最后一个探头是药物喷头,在再次使用激光打开感染细胞的同时,药物喷头直接向感染部位注入药物。

这个技术现在看起来还不太成熟,但是如果有一天能成功的话,就可以彻底消灭人体内的 HIV 病毒。是的,治愈艾滋病,这是每个 HIV 研究者的梦想——对我们来说,就是用激光来治愈艾滋病。

谢谢大家。

Lecture 6　The Next Outbreak？ We're Not Ready

下一次疫情暴发，我们准备好了吗？

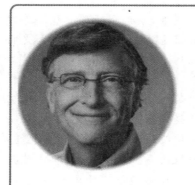

　　比尔·盖茨（Bill Gates），美国著名企业家、软件工程师和慈善家。1975年与好友保罗·艾伦一起创办了微软公司。2017年，他连续第24年蝉联美国首富宝座。2015年2月，比尔·盖茨获"2014全球最受尊敬的男人"称号。2016年1月，比尔·盖茨获IT与创新基金会评选的"卢德奖"提名。

　　比尔·盖茨一直致力于慈善事业。他创建了比尔与梅琳达·盖茨基金会，这是美国规模最大的慈善基金会。他曾宣布，自己不会从政，数百亿美元的巨额财富会捐献给社会，不会作为遗产留给子孙。2005年，比尔·盖茨被英国女王伊丽莎白二世授予荣誉爵士勋章，此勋章主要用于表彰盖茨与妻子梅琳达为消除英联邦及其他发展中国家的贫困状况、提高当地百姓的健康水平所做出的努力。2010年1月，比尔和梅琳达·盖茨在达沃斯论坛媒体发布会上表示，比尔和梅琳达·盖茨基金会将会在未来十年之内为世界上最贫穷的地区提供疫苗研究、开发与应用的支持。

1   When I was a kid, the disaster we worried about most was a nuclear war. That's why we had a barrel like this down in our basement, filled with cans of food and water. When the nuclear attack came, we were supposed to go downstairs, hunker down, and eat out of that barrel.

2   Today the greatest risk of global *catastrophe*①doesn't look like this. Instead, it looks like this. If anything kills over 10 million people in the next few decades, it's most likely to be a highly infectious virus rather than a war. Not missiles, but *microbes*②. Now, part of the reason for this is that we've invested a huge amount in nuclear *deterrents*③. But we've actually invested very little in a system to stop an epidemic. We're not ready for the next epidemic.

3   Let's look at Ebola. I'm sure all of you read about it in the newspaper, lots of tough challenges. I followed it carefully through the case analysis tools we use to track *polio*④*eradication*⑤. And as you look at what went on, the problem wasn't that there was a

1   在我小的时候，人们最担心的灾难是核战争。所以我们会在地下室里放上这样一个大桶，里面装满了罐头食物和水。当核战争爆发时，我们可以走进地下室，蹲下身子，靠桶里的食物维生。

2   现在，全球性灾难的最大危机看起来并非如此。相反，它是这样的。如果有什么东西会在未来几十年杀死上千万人，那么最有可能的是具有高度传染性的病毒而不是战争。不是导弹，而是微生物。导致这个灾难的部分原因是我们在核威慑力量上投入巨大，但在建立一个预防疫情的系统上却投入甚微。对于下一次疫情的爆发，我们并没有做好准备。

3   让我们来看一下埃博拉病毒。我相信大家都曾在报纸上读到过关于这个病毒的新闻。对此，我们面临着重重挑战。利用追踪消灭脊髓灰质炎的案例分析工具，我仔细追踪了埃博拉的发

---

① catastrophe *n.* 灾难
② microbe *n.* 微生物
③ deterrent *n.* 威慑力，震慑力
④ polio *n.* 小儿麻痹症；脊髓灰质炎
⑤ eradication *n.* 根除

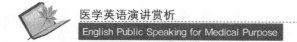

system that didn't work well enough; the problem was that we didn't have a system at all.

展。随着对疫情发展的关注，你会发现，问题并不在于我们的系统运营不善，而是我们根本没有这样一个系统。

4   In fact, there's some pretty obvious key missing pieces. We didn't have a group of *epidemiologists*①ready to go, who would have gone, seen what the disease was, seen how far it had spread. The case reports came in on paper. It was very delayed before they were put online and they were extremely inaccurate. We didn't have a medical team ready to go. We didn't have a way of preparing people. Now, *Médecins Sans Frontières*②did a great job *orchestrating*③volunteers. But even so, we were far slower than we should have been getting the thousands of workers into these countries. And a large epidemic would require us to have hundreds of thousands of workers. There was no one there to look at treatment approaches. No one to look at the diagnostics. No one to figure out what tools should be used. As an example, we could have taken the blood of survivors, processed it, and put that *plasma*④back in people to protect them. But that was never tried.

4   事实上，我们可以看到一些很明显的不足。例如，我们并没有一群准备充分的流行病学家，他们本应该去疫区观察疫情，关注疾情传播范围。关于病例的报道是从报纸传来的，网上看到的信息都是严重滞后且不准确的。我们没有一个准备充分的医护小组。我们没有设法让人们严阵以待。目前，无国界医生组织做了很多工作来动员志愿者。但即使如此，我们调动数千名工作者进入疫区的速度还远不能令人满意。而大型疫情需要调动数十万名工作者。但是，我们没有人去研究治疗方案，没有人去研究诊断方法，也没有人去解决该使用什么工具的问题。比如，我们本可以从幸存者身上提取血液，加工处理，然后再将血浆注入人们体内以保护他们。但是这个方法从来没有人试过。

---

①   epidemiologist *n.* 流行病学家
②   Médecins Sans Frontières 无国界医生组织
③   orchestrate *v.* 组织；策划
④   plasma *n.* 血浆

5   So there was a lot that was missing. And these things are really a global failure. The WHO is funded to monitor epidemics, but not to do these things I talked about. Now, in the movies it's quite different. There's a group of handsome epidemiologists ready to go, they move in, they save the day, but that's just pure Hollywood.

6   The failure to prepare could allow the next epidemic to be dramatically more *devastating*① than Ebola. Let's look at the progression of Ebola over this year. About 10,000 people died, and nearly all were in the three West African countries. There's three reasons why it didn't spread more. The first is that there was a lot of heroic work by the health workers. They found the people and they prevented more infections. The second is the nature of the virus. Ebola does not spread through the air. And by the time you're *contagious*②, most people are so sick that they're *bedridden*③. Third, it didn't get into many urban areas. And that was just luck. If it had gotten into a lot more urban areas, the case numbers would have been much larger.

5   因此,我们有很多事情没有做。而这实际上是全球性的失败。世界卫生组织的建立是用来监控流行病的,并不是来完成我刚才说的这些工作的。但是在电影里,情况完全不同。那里有一群英俊的流行病学家们时刻准备着。他们进入疫区,拯救了世界,但这仅仅是纯好莱坞的剧情。

6   如果我们没有做好充分的准备,下一次疫情将比埃博拉更具杀伤力。让我们来看看过去一年中埃博拉的发展。大约有1万人死亡,几乎都来自三个西非国家。有三个原因使得疫情没有在更大范围内传播。首先,医务工作者们做出了了不起的贡献。他们找到被感染者并阻止了疫情的传播。其次是病毒的本性。埃博拉并不会通过空气传播。等到你有传染力时,大多数人都已经生病并卧床不起。第三,病毒并没有传播到城区。这纯属幸运。如果它传播到城区,那么死亡人数要超出许多。

---

①　devastating *adj.* 毁坏性的;灾难性的
②　contagious *adj.* 有传染性的
③　bedridden *adj.* 长期卧床不起的

7   So next time, we might not be so lucky. You can have a virus where people feel well enough while they're infectious that they get on a plane or they go to a market. The source of the virus could be a natural epidemic like Ebola, or it could be *bioterrorism*①. So there are things that would literally make things a thousand times worse.

8   In fact, let's look at a model of a virus spread through the air, like the Spanish Flu back in 1918. So here's what would happen: It would spread throughout the world very, very quickly. And you can see over 30 million people died from that epidemic. So this is a serious problem. We should be concerned.

9   But in fact, we can build a really good response system. We have the benefits of all the science and technology that we talk about here. We've got cell phones to get information from the public and get information out to them. We have satellite maps where we can see where people are and where they're moving. We have advances in biology that should dramatically change the *turnaround*②time to look at a pathogen and be able to make drugs

7   下次我们不一定还会如此幸运。有些人被传染上病毒时自我感觉良好,但当他们去坐飞机或者去市场的时候已经具有传染性了。病毒的来源可能是像埃博拉这样的天然传染源,也有可能是生物恐怖主义。所以有的病毒会让疫情惨上一千倍。

8   现在,让我们来看一个病毒在空气中传播的模型,比如1918年的西班牙流感。情况是这样的:它会以非常非常快的速度传遍整个世界。你会看到超过3 000万人死于这个疾病。因此这是个严重的问题。我们必须予以关注。

9   但实际上,我们可以建立一个相当好的反应系统。我们可以利用所有发展至今的科学技术。我们有手机,可以从公众处获取信息,然后将信息反馈给他们。我们有卫星地图,可以看到人们在哪里,将向哪里移动。我们在生物学上取得了进展,可以大幅缩短找到病原体的时间,研制出适用于该病原体的药物和疫苗。

---

① bioterrorism *n.* 生物恐怖主义
② turnaround *n.* 周转;转机

and vaccines that fit for that pathogen. So we can have tools, but those tools need to be put into an overall global health system. And we need preparedness.

所以我们是有工具的,但是这些工具需要被纳入一个完整的全球卫生系统当中。而且我们需要做好准备应对疫情。

10　The best lessons, I think, on how to get prepared are again, what we do for war. For soldiers, we have full-time, waiting to go. We have *reserves*①that can scale us up to large numbers. NATO has a mobile unit that can *deploy*②very rapidly. NATO does a lot of war games to check. Are people well trained? Do they understand about fuel and *logistics*③and the same radio frequencies? So they are absolutely ready to go. So those are the kinds of things we need to deal with an epidemic.

10　我认为,要学习如何做好准备应对疫情,最好的榜样还是来自备战。士兵们是全天候、时刻准备着投入战争的。我们有预备军人,可以扩大备战人口的规模。北约组织有一个机动小组可以快速调动。北约组织开展了很多的军事演习来确认:士兵们是否得到了良好的训练? 他们是否了解燃油、后勤补给和相同的无线电频率? 因此,他们完全准备充分。所以,这也是应对疫情时我们需要做的。

11　What are the key pieces? First, we need strong health systems in poor countries. That's where mothers can give birth safely, kids can get all their vaccines. But, also where we'll see the outbreak very early on. We need a medical reserve corps: lots of people who've got the training and background who are ready to go,

11　那么,要点在哪里? 首先,我们需要在贫穷国家建立发达的卫生系统。这样母亲们可以安全地生下宝宝。孩子们可以接种疫苗。我们也可以在早期发现疫情的爆发。我们需要一个后备医疗部队,拥有大量接受过医疗训练、具有医疗背景、具备专业知识、随

---

①　reserve *n.* 预备队

②　deploy *v.* 部署;调配

③　logistics *n.* 物流;军事后勤

with the *expertise*①. And then we need to pair those medical people with the military, taking advantage of the military's ability to move fast, do logistics and secure areas. We need to do simulations, *germ*②games, not war games, so that we see where the holes are. The last time a germ game was done in the United States was back in 2001, and it didn't go so well. So far the score is germs：1, people：0. Finally, we need lots of advanced R&D in areas of vaccines and diagnostics. There are some big breakthroughs, like the *Adeno-associated virus*③, that could work very, very quickly.

时准备出发的工作人员。然后我们需要军队来配合医护人员,利用军队快速移动的能力来开展后勤保障和安保工作。我们需要做情景模拟,进行细菌演习而不是军事演习,这样我们可以发现漏洞在哪里。上一次的细菌演习是2001年在美国进行的,结果并不好。到目前为止,细菌得1分,人类得0分。最后,我们需要在疫苗和诊断学领域做大量前沿的研发工作。在某些方面,比如对腺相关病毒的研究,我们已经取得了一些重大的突破,这些研究成果很快会被运用到实践中。

12   Now I don't have an exact budget for what this would cost, but I'm quite sure it's very modest compared to the potential harm. The World Bank estimates that if we have a worldwide flu epidemic, global wealth will go down by over three trillion dollars and we'd have millions and millions of deaths. These investments offer significant benefits beyond just being ready for the epidemic. The primary healthcare, the R&D, those things would reduce global health *inequity*④and make the

12   现在,对于所需的花费,我并没有一个准确的预算。但我非常确定的是,同潜在的危害相比,这个金额不值一提。据世界银行预测,如果全球性流感爆发,全球经济损失将会超过3万亿美元,而且我们将失去数百万的生命。这些投资不仅仅让我们做好准备应对疫情,还能给我们带来巨大的好处。基础医疗卫生和医疗研发工作会促进全球健康的平衡发

---

①   expertise *n.* 专长;专门技能
②   germ *n.* 细菌
③   Adeno-associated virus *n.* 腺相关病毒
④   inequity *n.* 不公平,不公正

world more just as well as more safe.

展,会让我们的世界更美好更安全。

13   So I think this should absolutely be a priority. There's no need to panic. We don't have to hoard cans of spaghetti or go down into the basement. But we need to get going, because time is not on our side.

13　所以我认为这绝对是重中之重。没有必要恐慌。我们不需要储藏罐装的意大利面,也不需要躲进地下室。但是我们需要奋起直追,因为在时间上我们不占优势。

14   In fact, if there's one positive thing that can come out of the Ebola epidemic, it's that it can serve as an early warning, a wake-up call, to get ready. If we start now, we can be ready for the next epidemic. Thank you.

14　事实上,如果说埃博拉病毒能给我们带来什么正面影响的话,那就是,它可以作为一个预警,让我们觉醒并提前做好准备。如果我们现在开始行动的话,那么在下一次疫情暴发前,我们是可以准备好的。谢谢。

 演讲赏析

这是一篇有关政策问题的说服性演讲(persuasive speech on questions of policy)。2014 年埃博拉病毒的爆发给全世界人民敲响了警钟:疫情的防治迫在眉睫。比尔·盖茨希望通过演讲,说服大众齐心协力,利用一切可以利用的资源,从疫苗的研制和医疗工作者的培训开始,构建一个全球范围的卫生系统,为下一次疫情的爆发做好准备。

演讲用一个疑问句"*The next outbreak*?"及对其的否定回答"*We're not ready.*"作为标题,以一种开门见山的方式指出演讲的中心思想:对下一次疫情的爆发我们尚未做好充分的准备。这既震惊了听众(startle the audience),也成功吸引了他们的注意力(arouse the interest of the audience)。

在演讲的正文部分,演讲者采用了问题—成因—出路(problem-cause-solution)的方法来组织文章结构:首先提出问题,然后分析问题产生的原因和危害,最后提出解决问题的方法。

演讲第一部分(1~2段),演讲者用自己的经历(personal experience)开头,用大罐子(object)作为视觉辅助手段,激起听众对儿时的回忆,将听众与演讲内容关联起来(relate to the audience)。同时,通过对比的手段,演讲者提出问题:全球性灾难的最大问题是疫情的爆发,而我们尚未准备好。

演讲第二部分(3~5段),演讲者以埃博拉病毒为例(example),论证了问题产生的原因:我们缺少一个完善的应对疫情的系统。

那么,疫情的危害究竟有多大呢? 在演讲的第三部分(6~8段),演讲者通过西班牙流感的例子(example)和死亡人数的数据(statistics)告诉我们:这是一个严重的问题,我们必须予以关注。

接下来(9~11段),演讲者进一步论证了解决问题的可能性和方法:我们可以利用科学技术的发展、学习战备的方法,从而建立一个完整的全球卫生系统。

演讲倒数第二段(12段),演讲者通过引用世界银行的数据(statistics),再一次重申预防疫情的重要性。

最后(13~14段),演讲者使用首尾呼应法(refer to the introduction)来结束全文,指出:我们不再需要躲进地下室,但一定要对疫情有所防备。演讲的结束语与开篇语互相呼应,使得听众感受到演讲的完整性和一致性。

整篇演讲层层递进,运用了大量的例证和数据来论证观点;采用了简单而不失生动的PPT和实物来进行视觉辅助;语言清晰易懂,多处使用排比(parallelism)、头韵(alliteration)和对照(antithesis)等修辞手法来增强文章的感染力,是一篇非常成功的演讲。

精彩加油站

Plague Doctor in the 17th Century
17 世纪的瘟疫医生

精彩视频

In Italy, 1656—1657 devastating outbreaks of bubonic plague in Naples, Rome, and Genoa, killed approximately 200,000 - 400,000 people. It's unknown where this deadly plague originated, but it's said to have spread from Naples where restrictions and precautions were nonexistent.

In these cities, plague doctors were hired to treat plague patients especially for the poor who could not afford treatment. The doctors' costume was designed to protect them from what was thought of as evil smells or bad air, which was seen as the cause of infection at the time. This is now known as the medically obsolete miasma theory.

In reality the plague was caused by the bacterium Yersinia pestis, which exists in fleas found on rats. The infected would have flu symptoms followed by swollen and painful lymph nodes, gangrene, vomiting of blood, with death following within a week from infection.

Some historians point to Charles de

1656 年到 1657 年的意大利，极具毁灭性的黑死病在那不勒斯、罗马和热内亚全面爆发，20 万到 40 万人因此丧生。这种致命疾病的来源至今不详，但据说是从那不勒斯传过来的，因为那里没有任何限制和预防措施。

在这些城市，瘟疫医生被雇来治疗那些被瘟疫感染的病人，尤其是那些没钱看病的穷人。医生所穿的服装是特别设计的，目的是保护他们免受所谓的"邪恶气味"或"毒气"的传染。这些气味在当时被当作是感染源。现在我们把这归于医学上已过时的毒气理论。

事实上，这次瘟疫是由一种叫鼠疫杆菌的细菌引起的，这种细菌存活于老鼠身上的跳蚤里。被感染的病人会表现出流感症状，随后会出现淋巴结肿痛、坏疽和吐血，感染一周内就会死亡。

一些历史学家指出，查尔斯·

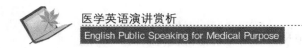

Lorme as the inventor of the costume, which was modeled after soldier's armor. The most striking feature was a bird beak-like mask with crystal glasses. The mask was more than aesthetic and acted as a respirator filled with dried flowers or spices, which the doctor breathed through, protecting them from contagions.

The doctor would also wear a long Moroccan leather gown that tucked into the mask to prevent contact with the patient. And the surface was waxed to prevent miasmas sticking to the surface. A friar named Father Antara Maria de San Vanna Bantora observed that those who worked in the plague house, while wearing the waxy robe did not catch the disease. He noted that it stopped fleas nesting on the person and was therefore close to discovering the true reason behind the plague. Unfortunately, he discounted the fleas as merely an annoyance rather than carriers of the disease and furthermore as the clothing didn't protect the wearer from miasmas. He would discount the value of waxed robes as well.

The doctors would also wear gloves, boots and a wide brimmed hat to show his profession and hold a wand or cane to examine and issue instruction without touching the patient.

德洛姆模仿士兵的盔甲，发明了医生制服。这种服装最引人注目的特点就是由水晶玻璃制成的鸟嘴状的面具。这种设计不仅仅是出于艺术的考量，还起到了防毒面具的作用。面具里装满了干花或香料，可以过滤医生呼吸的空气，保护他们免受传染。

医生还会穿一件摩洛哥式的长皮袍。皮袍的帽子被塞入面具里面，以防止医生同病人直接接触。皮袍的表面涂了一层蜡，以防止毒气附着在皮袍上。一位叫安塔拉的修士发现，那些穿了涂蜡长袍在瘟疫病房工作的人都没有被感染上疫病。因此，他指出长袍可以阻止跳蚤在人身上安家，这个结论已经很接近瘟疫的真正原因了。不幸的是，他低估了跳蚤，仅仅把它当作讨厌的东西，而不是病菌的携带者；而且他还认为衣服并不能保护穿着者免受毒气的侵害。就这样，他也低估了涂蜡长袍的作用。

医生们还需要戴手套、穿长靴和戴宽檐帽，以表明自己的职业。他们还会用手杖或拐棍来给病人做检查和下指令，这样他们就不会直接接触到病人了。

Methods of treatment for the miasma, which was really the plague，were ineffective. Remedies included bloodletting and the use of leeches on the affected areas. Prescriptions of toads or spiders were also given to absorb the bad air. The plague doctor's appearance was quite terrifying for patients，as it was a sign of impending death and they were kept out of the way of the public due to the nature of their profession.

这种所谓的毒气实际上是瘟疫，所以针对毒气的治疗方法并没有效果。当时的治疗手段包括放血和将水蛭投放至被感染区域。也有处方中用蟾蜍和蜘蛛来吸收毒气。瘟疫医生的到来对于病人来说是十分可怕的，因为这意味着死亡即将来临。因其职业特点，民众对瘟疫医生都是避而远之。

Lecture 7   Alzheimer's Is Not Normal Aging—and We Can Cure It

阿尔茨海默病不是正常衰老的必然结果
——我们可以治愈它

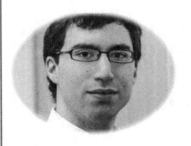

　　萨缪尔·科赫恩（Samuel Cohen）是英国剑桥大学圣约翰学院生物物理化学方向的一名研究员，本科至研究生阶段皆在剑桥大学开展学习和研究工作。同时，他也是波士顿咨询公司（BCG）伦敦办公室的一名咨询顾问，擅长健康保健领域以及技术与媒体领域的咨询工作。这些年来，他致力于对神经退化性疾病的研究，以第一作者或合作者的身份取得的研究成果（论文、著作和专利）超过 20 项。最近他以第一作者的身份发表了一篇受到广泛关注的论文，在文中展示了研究者们在治疗阿尔茨海默病方面的重大突破。

1   In the year 1901, a woman called Auguste was taken to a medical asylum in Frankfurt. Auguste was *delusional*①and couldn't remember even the most basic details of her life. Her doctor was called Alois. Alois didn't know how to help Auguste, but he watched over her until, sadly, she passed away in 1906. After she died, Alois performed an *autopsy*②and found strange *plaques*③and *tangles*④in Auguste's brain—the likes of which he'd never seen before.

2   Now here's the even more striking thing. If Auguste had instead been alive today, we could offer her no more help than Alois was able to 114 years ago. Alois was Dr. Alois Alzheimer. And Auguste Deter was the first patient to be diagnosed with what we now call *Alzheimer's disease*⑤. Since 1901, medicine has advanced greatly. We've discovered *antibiotics*⑥and *vaccines*⑦to protect us from infections, many treatments for cancer, *antiretrovirals*⑧for HIV, *statins*⑨for heart disease and much more. But we've made essentially no progress at

1   1901 年，一个叫奥古斯特的女人被带到了法兰克福的一家医疗收容所。她患有妄想症，并且连生活中常见的事情都记不住。她的医生叫爱罗斯。爱罗斯不知如何治疗奥古斯特，但一直关注着她的病情，直到 1906 年奥古斯特不幸去世。她死后，爱罗斯对她进行了尸检，在她的大脑中发现了之前从未见过的奇怪的斑块和纤维缠结。

2   还有一件事更令人震惊。如果奥古斯特生活在今天，我们能够给予她的帮助也不会比 114 年前爱罗斯为她做的更多。爱罗斯就是爱罗斯·阿尔茨海默医生。而奥古斯特·迪特是第一个被诊断为患有阿尔茨海默病的病人。1901 年至今，医学研究获得了巨大的发展。我们发明了抗生素和疫苗以使我们不被感染，找到了许多方法来治疗癌症，研制了抗反转录病毒药物来治疗艾滋

① delusional *adj.* 妄想的
② autopsy *n.* 尸体解剖
③ plaque *n.* 斑块
④ tangle *n.* 缠结
⑤ Alzheimer's disease *n.* 阿尔茨海默病
⑥ antibiotics *n.* 抗生素
⑦ vaccine *n.* 疫苗
⑧ antiretrovirals *n.* 抗反转录病毒药物
⑨ statin *n.* 抑制素，斯达汀（药物名）

all in treating Alzheimer's disease.

病，开发了他汀类药物来对抗心脏病等等。但是在治疗阿尔茨海默病方面，我们基本上没有什么进展。

3 I'm part of a team of scientists who has been working to find a cure for Alzheimer's for over a decade. So I think about this all the time. Alzheimer's now affects 40 million people worldwide. But by 2050, it will affect 150 million people—which, by the way, will include many of you. If you're hoping to live to be 85 or older, your chance of getting Alzheimer's will be almost one in two. In other words, odds are you'll spend your golden years either suffering from Alzheimer's or helping to look after a friend or loved one with Alzheimer's. Already in the United States alone, Alzheimer's care costs 200 billion dollars every year. One out of every five Medicare dollars get spent on Alzheimer's. It is today the most expensive disease, and costs are projected to increase five-fold by 2050, as the baby boomer generation ages.

3 我所在的科学家团队已经花了十几年时间来寻找治疗阿尔茨海默病的方法。所以我一直都在思考这个问题。目前全世界有4 000万阿尔茨海默病患者。但是到2050年，这一数字将增至1亿5 000万——在座的很多人都可能包括在内。如果你想要活到85岁以上，那么患上阿尔茨海默病的概率将达到50%。换句话说，晚年的你要么会饱受阿尔茨海默病的折磨，要么得照顾患有阿尔茨海默病的朋友或者爱人。目前，仅仅在美国，每年用来治疗阿尔茨海默病的费用就高达2 000亿美元。每5美元的医疗保险费用中，就有1美元用在了阿尔茨海默病患者的身上。它是目前最昂贵的疾病，到2050年，治疗费用预计会增加5倍，因为在婴儿潮时期出生的人，那时都将步入老年。

4 It may surprise you that, put simply, Alzheimer's is one of the biggest medical and social challenges of our generation. But we've

4 简单点说，虽然听起来有些

done relatively little to *address*①it. Today，of the top 10 causes of death worldwide，Alzheimer's is the only one we cannot prevent，cure or even slow down. We understand less about the science of Alzheimer's than other diseases because we've invested less time and money into researching it. The US government spends 10 times more every year on cancer research than on Alzheimer's despite the fact that Alzheimer's costs us more and causes a similar number of deaths each year as cancer.

5   The lack of resources stems from a more fundamental cause：a lack of awareness. Because here's what few people know but everyone should：Alzheimer's is a disease，and we can cure it. For most of the past 114 years，everyone，including scientists，mistakenly confused Alzheimer's with aging. We thought that becoming *senile*②was a normal and inevitable part of getting old. But we only have to look at a picture of a healthy aged brain compared to the brain of an Alzheimer's patient to see the real physical damage caused by this

不可思议,但阿尔茨海默病可能是我们这一代人面临的最大的医疗和社会挑战之一。然而,我们对它却基本没有采取什么行动。今天,在全世界导致死亡的十大因素中,阿尔茨海默病是唯一一个无法预防、治愈甚至控制的。相对于对其他疾病的了解,我们对阿尔茨海默病知之甚少,因为我们在研究这一疾病上所投入的时间和资金都相对较少。美国政府每年花费在癌症研究上的费用比花费在阿尔茨海默病研究上的要多 10 倍,尽管阿尔茨海默病的治疗花费其实更高,且每年造成的死亡人数几乎与癌症相等。

5   研究匮乏的一个主要原因是:人们对这种疾病不够重视。这是一个几乎无人知晓但本应人尽皆知的事实:阿尔茨海默病是一种疾病,并且我们可以治愈它。在过去的 114 年里,包括科学家在内的所有人都错误地把阿尔茨海默病和衰老混为一谈。我们认为年老糊涂是人在衰老后难以避免的样子。但是我们只需要将健康老年人的大脑图与阿尔茨海默病患者的大脑图进行对比,就会

---

① address *v.* 对付,解决
② senile *adj.* 衰老的,老年的

disease. As well as triggering severe loss of memory and mental abilities, the damage to the brain caused by Alzheimer's significantly reduces life expectancy and is always fatal.

发现这个疾病对大脑造成的真正的损伤。除了会严重导致记忆力和思维能力的丧失,阿尔茨海默病对大脑的伤害还会严重影响人的寿命,并且常常是致命的。

6　Remember Dr. Alzheimer found strange plaques and tangles in Auguste's brain a century ago. For almost a century, we didn't know much about these. Today we know they're made from *protein*①*molecules*②. You can imagine a protein molecule as a piece of paper that normally folds into an elaborate piece of *origami*③. There are spots on the paper that are sticky. And when it folds correctly, these sticky bits end up on the inside. But sometimes things go wrong, and some sticky bits are on the outside. This causes the protein molecules to stick to each other, forming *clumps*④that eventually become large plaques and tangles. That's what we see in the brains of Alzheimer's patients.

6　回想一下一百年前阿尔茨海默医生在奥古斯特大脑里发现的那些奇怪的斑块和纤维缠结吧。一个世纪过去了,我们并不比当年了解的更多。今天,我们知道那些斑块和纤维缠结是由蛋白质分子构成的。你可以把一个蛋白质分子想象成一张纸,而这张纸被折叠成一个精细的手工作品。这张纸上有一些黏糊糊的点。当这张纸被正确折叠时,这些有黏性的点被锁在了内部。但有些时候出错了,一些有黏性的点就会暴露在外部。这导致一些蛋白质分子互相粘连,形成了凝块,最终发展成为大的斑块和纤维缠结。这就是我们在阿尔茨海默病患者大脑中看到的东西。

7　We've spent the past 10 years at the

7　我们花了十年的时间在剑桥

---

① protein *n.* 蛋白质
② molecule *n.* 分子
③ origami *n.* 折纸工艺
④ clump *n.* 团,堆,凝块

University of Cambridge trying to understand how this ***malfunction***①works. There are many steps，and identifying which step to try to block is complex—like ***defusing***②a bomb. Cutting one wire might do nothing. Cutting others might make the bomb explore. We have to find the right step to block，and then create a drug that does it.

大学研究并试图理解这种病变是如何产生的。病变有很多阶段，而确定在哪一步可以阻止病变是非常复杂的——就像拆弹一样。切断一根线也许什么都不会发生。切断别的线，炸弹可能就会爆炸。我们必须要找到阻断病变的关键环节，然后发明一种药物来实现这个阻断。

8　Until recently，we for the most part have been cutting wires and hoping for the best. But now we've got together a diverse group of people—medics，biologists，geneticists，chemists，physicists，engineers and mathematicians. And together，we've managed to identify a critical step in the process and are now testing a new class of drugs which would specifically block this step and stop the disease.

8　直到不久前，我们仍在花费大力气去尝试一根根地切线，并期待能找到那个最关键的环节。但现在，我们把一群不同背景的人汇集在一起——医生、生物学家、遗传学家、化学家、物理学家、工程师和数学家。通过合作，我们已经成功锁定了病变中的一个关键环节，并且正在测试一批新的药物来阻断该环节，控制住病情。

9　Now let me show you some of our latest results. No one outside of our lab has seen these yet. Let's look at some videos of what happened when we tested these new drugs in worms. So these are healthy worms, and you can see they're moving around normally. These

9　现在我来给大家展示一下我们最新的研究成果。目前，除了我们实验室的人，还没有旁人看到过这些。让我们通过短片来看一下这批新药在虫子身上测试的结果。（左边）这些是健康的虫

---

① malfunction *n.*（人体器官）机能失常
② defuse *v.* 拆除（引爆物）

worms, on the other hand, have protein molecules sticking together inside them—like humans with Alzheimer's. And you can see they're clearly sick. But if we give our new drugs to these worms at an early stage, then we see that they're healthy, and they live a normal lifespan. This is just an initial positive result, but research like this shows us that Alzheimer's is a disease that we can understand and we can cure.

子,你们可以看到它们能够正常地蠕动。而(中间)这些虫子体内有一些蛋白质分子粘连在一起,就像是患有阿尔茨海默病的病人。很明显,它们生病了。但是如果在患病早期给这些虫子使用我们的新药,我们可以看到(右边)这些虫子康复了,并且可以活到正常的寿命。这只是研究初期一个较为乐观的结果,但这样的研究表明阿尔茨海默病是一个我们能够了解并且可以治愈的疾病。

10　After 114 years of waiting, there's finally real hope for what can be achieved in the next 10 or 20 years. But to grow that hope, to finally beat Alzheimer's, we need help. This isn't about scientists like me—it's about you. We need you to raise awareness that Alzheimer's is a disease and that if we try, we can beat it. In the case of other diseases, patients and their families have led the charge for more research and put pressure on governments, the *pharmaceutical*① industry, scientists and regulators. That was essential for advancing treatment for HIV in the late 1980s. Today, we see that same drive to beat cancer. But Alzheimer's patients are often unable to speak up for themselves. And their families,

10　在等待了 114 年之后,我们终于对未来 10 年至 20 年的研究进展有了真正的期待。但是想要梦想成真,想要彻底战胜阿尔茨海默病,我们需要帮助。这种帮助不是来自像我一样的科学家,而是来自你们。我们需要大家增进对阿尔茨海默病的了解,并认识到如果我们努力,就可以打败它。就其他疾病而言,是患者和家属促成了更多的研究,他们给政府、制药企业、科学家和管理者施加了压力。在 20 世纪 80 年代后期,这种努力对于推进艾滋病的治疗至关重要。今天,在对抗癌症方面,我们也看到了相同的

———————————

①　pharmaceutical *adj.* 制药的

the hidden victims, caring for their loved ones night and day, are often too worn out to go out and advocate for change. So, it really is down to you. Alzheimer's isn't, for the most part, a genetic disease. Everyone with a brain is at risk. Today, there are 40 million patients like Auguste, who can't create the change they need for themselves. Help speak up for them, and help demand a cure.

推动力。但是阿尔茨海默病患者常常不能为自己发声。而他们的家人，那些潜在的受害者，因为要没日没夜地照顾他们所爱的人，也筋疲力尽而无力站出来推动这种变革。所以，这有赖于你们。阿尔茨海默病大多不是由遗传因素导致的。每个有大脑的人都有患此病的风险。如今，有4 000万像奥古斯特那样的病人无法推进这场他们所需要的变革。请为他们发声，帮助他们推动治疗阿尔茨海默病的研究。

11 Thank you.

11 谢谢大家。

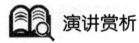 演讲赏析

这是一篇有关政策问题的说服性演讲(persuasive speech on questions of policy)。演讲者按照"问题—成因—出路"(problem-cause-solution)的方法展开论证，号召人们增进对阿尔茨海默病的关注和了解，推动阿尔茨海默病的研究。

在演讲的开头部分，演讲者以讲故事的方式(tell a story)介绍了世界上第一例阿尔茨海默病患者被发现的始末，然后表达了一个令听众震惊(startle the audience)的观点：如果奥古斯特生活在今天，我们能够给予她的帮助也不会比114年前爱罗斯为她做的更多。在此基础上，演讲者提出了需要论证的主要问题(problem)，即本演讲的第一个主要观点(first main point)：在治疗阿尔茨海默病方面，我们基本上没有什么进展。

在演讲的主体部分，首先，演讲者罗列了多项数据(multiple statistics)，包括全世界阿尔茨海默病患者人数，85岁以上人群患阿尔茨海默病的概率，美国每年

用来治疗阿尔茨海默病的花费等等,进一步说明了问题的严重性,并一针见血地指出了问题存在的主要原因(cause),即本演讲的第二个主要观点(second main point):人们对这种疾病不够重视。随后,演讲者两次使用了打比方的修辞手法(simile and metaphor):一次将蛋白质分子比喻成一张纸,生动地说明了阿尔茨海默病的成因;一次将阻断病变的过程比喻成拆弹的过程,告诉听众推进阿尔茨海默病研究的困难之处。而这两处说解,为听众提供了了解阿尔茨海默病的必要知识,为号召听众采取行动(to gain immediate action)做好了准备。

在演讲的结尾部分,演讲者通过视频呈现了其团队研究的最新成果,表明阿尔茨海默病是一个我们能够了解并且可以治愈的疾病,并在此基础上提出了推进阿尔茨海默病研究的办法(solution),即本演讲的第三个主要观点(third main point):请大家增进对阿尔茨海默病的了解,像20世纪80年代推进艾滋病研究一样给政府、制药企业、科学家和管理者施加压力,替阿尔茨海默病患者及其家属发声,帮助他们推动这场变革。

纵观整个演讲,演讲者语言朴实,论证有理有据(using evidence),声调抑扬顿挫(vocal variety),停顿(pause)恰当,眼神交流(eye contact)自然真挚,使演讲充满了感染力和说服力。

 精彩加油站

Weekly Address:Celebrating Fifty Years of Medicare and Medicaid
美国总统奥巴马每周演讲:
庆祝医疗保险和医疗补助制度实施50周年

精彩视频

Hi, everybody. This week, there was a big birthday you might have missed. Medicare and Medicaid turned 50 years old. And that's something worth celebrating.

大家好!本周,你们可能错过了一个重大的节日。医疗保险和医疗补助制度已经实施50年了。这是一件值得庆贺的事情。

If one of the best measures of a country is how it treats its more vulnerable citizens—seniors, the poor, the sick—then America has a lot to be proud of. Think about it. Before Social Security, too many seniors lived in poverty. Before Medicare, only half had some form of health insurance. Before Medicaid, parents often had no help covering the cost of care for a child with a disability.

But as Americans, we declared that our citizens deserve a basic measure of security and dignity. And today, the poverty rate for seniors is less than half of what it was fifty years ago. Every American over 65 has access to affordable health care. And today, we're finally finishing the job—since I signed the Affordable Care Act into law, the uninsured rate for all Americans has fallen by about one-third.

These promises we made as a nation have saved millions of our own people from poverty and hardship, allowing us new freedom, new independence, and the chance to live longer, better lives. That's something to be proud of. It's heroic. These endeavors—these American endeavors—they didn't just make us a better country. They reaffirmed that we are a great country.

如果说衡量一个国家是否优秀的最佳标准之一是她如何对待老人、穷人、病人等弱势公民的话，美国在这一点上可以说是相当自豪的。大家回想一下。在社会保险制度实施之前，很多老人穷困潦倒。在医疗保险制度实施之前，全国仅有一半的人口有某种形式的医疗保险。在医疗补助制度实施以前，残疾儿童的父母只能独自承担照料病儿的费用。

但作为美国人，我们认为我们的公民应该享有基本的保障与尊严。今天，贫困老年人的比例只有50年前的一半不到。每个65岁以上的美国人都可以享受负担得起的医疗保险。现在这个任务终于完成了。自从我签署了《平价医疗法案》以后，全国未参保人数比例已经下降了约三分之一。

我们在国家层面所做出的这些承诺，已经让数百万民众脱离了贫困，让我们享有新的自由和自主，让我们有机会享受更长久、更优质的生活。这是值得我们骄傲的事情，是壮举。这些努力——我们美国人的努力——不仅让美国成为更优秀的国家，更让美国成为一个伟大的国家。

And a great country keeps the promises it makes. Today, we're often told that Medicare and Medicaid are in crisis. But that's usually a political excuse to cut their funding, privatize them, or phase them out entirely—all of which would undermine their core guarantee. The truth is, these programs aren't in crisis. Nor have they kept us from cutting our deficits by two-thirds since I took office. What is true is that every month, another 250,000 Americans turn 65 years old, and become eligible for Medicare. And we all deserve a health care system that delivers efficient, high-quality care. So to keep these programs strong, we'll have to make smart changes over time, just like we always have.

Today, we're actually proving that's possible. The Affordable Care Act has already helped secure Medicare's funding for another 13 years. The Affordable Care Act has saved more than nine million folks on Medicare 15 billion dollars on their prescription medicine. It has expanded Medicaid to help cover 12.8 million more Americans, and to help more seniors live independently. And we're moving our health care system toward models that reward the quality of the care you receive, not the quantity of care you receive. That means healthier Americans and a healthier federal

一个伟大的国家总是坚守她的承诺。现在,我们经常听到有人说医疗保险和医疗补助制度危机重重。但这通常只是有些人想要减少医疗资金投入、对医疗实行私有化,甚至完全推翻这一体系的政治借口而已,而所有的这些企图都会削弱医保和医补制度的核心保障能力。事实上,这些制度并未处在危机之中。且自我主政以来,这些政策也并未妨碍我们将财政赤字削减了三分之二。事实是,每个月都有25万美国人步入65岁,成为医疗保险的受益者。每个人都应该享有能够提供高效、优质服务的医保体系。因此,为了让这些政策更稳固,我们需要像以往一样,经受住时间的考验并做出明智的选择。

现在,我们正在证明这么做是可行的。《平价医疗法案》已经为今后13年的医疗保险资金来源提供了保障,也已经让900多万民众利用医疗保险在处方药支出上节约了150亿美元。该法案还使1 280万新增人群享受到了医疗补助,使更多的老年人能够独立生活。同时,我们正在改进医疗保险体系,使其模式更有利于民众享受到医疗服务的质量,而不是数量。这意味着未来美国人会更健康,我们的联邦预算也会更稳健。

budget.

Today, these programs are so fundamental to our way of life that it's easy to forget how hard people fought against them at the time. When FDR created Social Security, critics called it socialism. When JFK and LBJ worked to create Medicare, the cynics said it would take away our freedom. But ultimately, we came to see these programs for what they truly are—a promise that if we work hard, and play by the rules, we'll be rewarded with a basic measure of dignity, security, and the freedom to live our lives as we want.

It's a promise that previous generations made to us, and a promise that our generation has to keep.

Thanks, and have a great weekend.

今天，这些制度已经成为我们生活的基本组成部分，我们很容易忘记之前人们是如何强烈反对这些制度的。当罗斯福总统创立社会保障体系时，批评人士称他是社会主义者。当肯尼迪总统和约翰逊总统致力于建立医疗保险制度时，有人怀疑其会破坏我们的自由。但最终，我们都看到了这些制度真正的力量——这是一个承诺：只要努力工作，遵纪守法，我们就可以享有基本的尊严和保障，自由地过上我们想要的生活。

这是先辈向我们许下的诺言，而我们这代人应该继续遵守这个诺言。

谢谢大家，祝周末愉快！

Lecture 8   A Second Opinion on Developmental Disorders
关于学习障碍的新认识

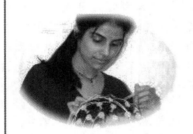

　　阿底提·香卡达斯（Aditi Shankardass）是一名神经科学家，她的学习经历横跨神经生理学、神经解剖学以及神经心理学三个学科，同时也在细胞神经科学和认知神经科学等不同的领域从事实验研究和临床工作。她目前是加州州立大学沟通障碍系神经生理实验室的负责人。她的研究重点为使用数字定量脑电图实时记录脑电活动，并进行分析，以更加精准地诊断儿童发育障碍。她也是全球神经科学基金会的理事以及 BBC《科学前沿》节目的顾问。

1   When I was 10 years old, a cousin of mine took me on a tour of his medical school. And as a special treat, he took me to the pathology lab and took a real human brain out of the jar and placed it in my hands. And there it was, the seat of human consciousness, the powerhouse of the human body, sitting in my hands. And that day I knew that when I grew up, I was going to become a brain doctor, scientist, something or the other.

2   Years later, when I finally grew up, my dream came true. And it was while I was doing my Ph. D. on the *neurological*①causes of *dyslexia*②in children that I encountered a startling fact that I'd like to share with you all today. It is estimated that one in six children, that's one in six children, suffer from some developmental disorder. This is a disorder that *retards*③mental development in the child and causes permanent mental *impairments*④. Which means that each and every one of you here today knows at least one child that is suffering from a developmental disorder.

3   But here's what really *perplexed*⑤me.

1   我十岁的时候，表哥带我去他就读的医学院。他特地带我去了病理实验室，从瓶子里拿出一个真正的人脑，放在我手里。就是它了，人类意识的来源，人体的能量源泉，就那样躺在我的手心里。从那天起，我就知道长大以后我不是会成为一名脑科医生，就是一名脑科学家，或者是做其他类似的工作。

2   多年以后，我长大成人，梦想成真。在攻读博士学位，研究儿童阅读障碍的神经因素的时候，我发现一个惊人的事实，这也是今天我想与你们分享的内容。据估算约有六分之一的儿童患有某种发育障碍，这种障碍会造成儿童心智发育滞后以及永久性心智损伤。也就是说，在座的各位肯定会认识至少一名患有发育障碍的儿童。

3   令我真正感到困惑的是，尽

① neurological *adj.* 神经学的
② dyslexia *n.* 读写障碍
③ retard *v.* 阻碍，减缓
④ impairment *n.* 缺陷，障碍
⑤ perplex *v.* 使……困惑

Despite the fact that each and every one of these disorders originates in the brain, most of these disorders are diagnosed solely on the basis of observable behavior. But diagnosing a brain disorder without actually looking at the brain is analogous to treating a patient with a heart problem based on their physical symptoms, without even doing an *ECG*①or a chest X-ray to look at the heart. It seemed so *intuitive*②to me. To diagnose and treat a brain disorder accurately, it would be necessary to look at the brain directly. Looking at behavior alone can miss a vital piece of the puzzle and provide an incomplete, or even a misleading, picture of the child's problems. Yet, despite all the advances in medical technology, the diagnosis of brain disorders in one in six children still remained so limited.

4　And then I came across a team at Harvard University that had taken one such advanced medical technology and finally applied it, instead of in brain research, towards diagnosing brain disorders in children. Their groundbreaking technology records the *EEG*③, or the electrical activity of the brain, in real time, allowing us to watch the brain as it performs various

管所有的发育障碍都源于大脑，但大多数障碍只能通过行为观察诊断。绕过大脑诊断脑部疾病，就好比不做心电图或胸部 X 光，只针对身体症状治疗心脏病。要准确诊断脑部疾病，必须直接检查大脑，这在我看来理所当然。只观察行为，就会错失重要信息，对疾病产生不完整，甚至错误的理解。尽管医学技术取得了很大进步，而面对发病率高达六分之一的儿童脑部疾病，我们的诊断方法却极为有限。

4　后来，我遇到了哈佛大学一个研究小组，他们已经研发出了这种先进的医疗技术，并把它应用到了诊断儿童脑部发育障碍中，而并不仅仅是脑部研究。这一创新的技术可以实时记录脑电图或者脑部电波活动，这样我们就可以在大脑执行不同功能时观察其活动，检测大脑在执行视

---

①　ECG（＝electrocardiogram）心电图

②　intuitive *adj.* 直觉的，直观的

③　EEG（＝electroencephalography）脑电图

functions and then detect even the slightest *abnormality*①in any of these functions: vision, attention, language, audition. A program called Brain Electrical Activity Mapping then *triangulates*②the source of that abnormality in the brain. And another program called Statistical Probability Mapping then performs mathematical calculations to determine whether any of these abnormalities are clinically significant, allowing us to provide a much more accurate neurological diagnosis of the child's symptoms. And so I became the head of *neurophysiology*③for the clinical arm of this team, and we're finally able to use this technology towards actually helping children with brain disorders. And I'm happy to say that I'm now in the process of setting up this technology here in India.

5   I'd like to tell you about one such child, whose story was also covered by ABC News. Seven-year-old Justin Senigar came to our clinic with this diagnosis of very severe *autism*④. Like many autistic children, his mind was locked inside his body. There were moments when he would actually space out for seconds at a time. And the doctors told his parents he was

觉、注意力、语言、听觉等活动时出现的哪怕是最最细微的异常情况。一个叫做 Brain Electrical Activity Mapping 的程序会用三角测量法确定脑部异常的根源。另外一个叫做 Statistical Probability Mapping 的程序可以用数学计算的方法,确定这些异常是否具有临床意义,以便于我们对儿童脑部疾病症状进行更加精确的神经诊断。于是,我成为这一神经生理学团队中临床分组的组长,成功地使用这一技术辅助诊断儿童脑部疾病。我很高兴地告诉大家,这一技术即将被印度引进使用。

5   我想分享一个患儿的经历,他的事情也曾被 ABC 新闻报道过。7 岁的贾斯汀·塞尼格来我们诊所时,已经被诊断为严重的自闭症。和许多自闭症患儿一样,他的思维被禁锢在身体内,时不时地发呆几秒钟。医生告诉他父母,他永远无法和他人正常交

① abnormality *n.* 反常,不正常
② triangulate *v.* 作三角测量
③ neurophysiology *n.* 神经生理机能
④ autism *n.* 自闭症

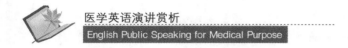
never going to be able to communicate or interact socially, and he would probably never have too much language.

流,甚至可能不太会说话。

6   When we used this groundbreaking EEG technology to actually look at Justin's brain, the results were startling. It turned out that Justin was almost certainly not autistic. He was suffering from brainseizures that were impossible to see with the naked eye, but that were actually causing symptoms that *mimicked*①those of autism. After Justin was given anti-seizure medication, the change in him was amazing. Within a period of 60 days, his vocabulary went from two to three words to 300 words. And his communication and social interaction were improved so dramatically that he was enrolled into a regular school and even became a *karate*②super champ.

6   我们使用新的脑电图技术研究了贾斯汀的脑部,结果令人吃惊:几乎可以肯定的是他并没有自闭症,他只是患有无法用肉眼察觉到的脑癫痫,而这种癫痫引起的症状与自闭症极为相似。在服用了抗癫痫药之后,贾斯汀病情明显改善。两个月后,他的词汇量从两三个扩大到了三百。沟通和社交能力也明显提高,不仅正常入学学习,还获得了空手道超级冠军。

7   Research shows that 50 percent of children, almost 50 percent of children diagnosed with autism are actually suffering from hidden brain seizures. These are the faces of the children that I have tested with stories just like Justin. All these children came to our clinic with a diagnosis of autism, attention *deficit*③disorder,

7   研究表明,约有50%被诊断为自闭症的儿童患有隐性脑癫痫。这些是我曾经检查过的孩子们的脸,他们和贾斯汀的病情相似。所有这些孩子都被诊断为自闭症、注意力缺乏症、智力发育迟缓、语言障碍。而脑电图显示,他

---

① mimick *v.* 模仿
② karate *n.* 空手道
③ deficit *n.* 不足,短缺

mental *retardation*①, language problems. Instead，our EEG scans revealed very specific problems hidden within their brains that couldn't possibly have been detected by their behavioral assessments. So these EEG scans enabled us to provide these children with a much more accurate neurological diagnosis and much more targeted treatment.

8　For too long now, children with developmental disorders have suffered from misdiagnosis while their real problems have gone undetected and left to worsen. And for too long, these children and their parents have suffered undue frustration and desperation. But we are now in a new era of neuroscience，one in which we can finally look directly at brain function in real time with no risks and no side effects，*non-invasively*②， and find the true source of so many disabilities in children.

9　So if I could inspire even a fraction of you in the audience today to share this pioneering diagnostic approach with even one parent whose child is suffering from a developmental disorder，then perhaps one more puzzle in one more brain will be solved. One more mind will be unlocked. And one more child who has been

们的脑部出了问题，可行为评估却无法发现。因此脑电图可以给这些孩子们提供更加准确的神经诊断，以便进行更加有的放矢的治疗。

8　长期以来，许多患有发育障碍的孩子被误诊，他们真正的病情却被忽视并恶化。长期以来，这些孩子以及他们的父母承受了太多无谓的沮丧与绝望。现在神经科学的新纪元已经到来，我们可以不用担心任何风险和副作用，实时无创地检查脑部功能，找到孩子们患病的根源。

9　也许今天我的演讲可以触动的仅仅是在座的一部分人，可只要你们和一位患儿的家长分享了这些信息，那么或许又一个孩子的脑部问题可以得到解决，又一个被禁锢的大脑可以被解放，又一个被误诊或未得到诊断的孩子

---

① retardation *n*. 迟滞，迟钝
② non-invasively *adv*. 无创伤地

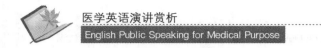

misdiagnosed or even undiagnosed by the system will finally realize his or her true potential while there's still time for his or her brain to recover. And all this by simply watching the child's brainwaves.

将最终发掘出自己的潜能,而那时他(她)的大脑还来得及恢复。要做到这一切很简单,你需要的仅仅是去看一眼孩子的脑电图。

10   Thank you.

10   谢谢!

 演讲赏析

人们对疾病的认知总是随着医学研究的飞速发展而不断更新。本篇演讲是一篇说服类演讲(persuasive speech),旨在说服听众接受一种新诊断方法——通过脑电波诊断儿童发展障碍。就演讲的组织方法(strategic order)而言,演讲者选用了动机序列法(motivated sequence)。首先,她结合自己成为脑科学家的经历,指出一个令人震惊的事实——发病率高达六分之一的儿童发展障碍,本质上属于脑部疾病;而一直以来,这种疾病却是通过观察行为来进行诊断的。这样的开头,成功地获得了观众的关注,让观众觉得这种疾病急需新的诊断方法。接下来,她提出应用脑电图技术可以更准确地诊断儿童发展障碍。为了便于听众理解,她选用了具体的病例(extended example),通过讲述一个患有癫痫却被误诊为自闭症的患儿贾斯汀的诊断及治疗过程:贾斯汀发育迟缓,一开始被误诊为自闭症,而在运用新的脑电图技术确诊为脑癫痫并服用抗癫痫药后,他的认知和学习能力有了极大的提高。这一具体病例描述了正确诊断给患儿带来的巨大变化,凸显新诊断方法的优点。最后一段里,演讲者更直接明了地对听众发出号召:希望听众可以与身边的患儿家长分享这些信息,以帮助更多有脑部问题的孩子得到正确诊断。

值得注意的是,由于面对的是普通听众而非专业人士,尽管信息量非常大,演讲者自始至终使用的都是日常词汇而非专业用语,比如在描述自闭症(autism)患儿情况的时候,她是这样形容的:"*his mind was locked inside his body.*"这样的描述让听众更加容易听懂接受。此外,演讲者还适当运用了统计数据(statistics)来令观众更加信服,如在谈到患病比例时,她提到约有六分之一的儿童患有某种发育障碍（*one in six children suffer from some developmental disorder*），另外约有 50%被诊断为自闭症的儿童患有隐性脑癫痫（*Research shows that 50 percent of children，almost 50 percent of children diagnosed with autism are actually suffering from hidden brain seizures*）。这样的两个统计数据，让听众对于患病儿童的比率有了更为直接清晰的了解。在演讲时，她还对这两个数据进行了重复，以强调患病儿童比例之高。

此外，演讲者还运用了重复（repetition）的修辞手法。如在第九段中，"*one more puzzle in one more brain will be solved*"，"*One more mind will be unlocked*"，"*And one more child who has been misdiagnosed or even undiagnosed by the system*"，这样的重复结构不仅增加了语言的节奏感（rhythm），还让演讲的结尾更具说服力。

这篇演讲，篇幅不长，却极为有效地传达了演讲者所要表达的信息：传统的行为诊断法不足以精确诊断儿童发展障碍，而通过脑电图进行神经诊断，从而更为准确地提供治疗，必将大大降低误诊率，给无数患儿带来希望。

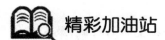

精彩加油站

The Best Gift I Ever Survived
我收到最好的礼物

精彩视频

Imagine，if you will—a gift. I'd like for you to picture it in your mind. It's not too big—about the size of a golf ball. So envision what it looks like all wrapped up. But before I show you what's inside, I will tell you, it's going to do incredible things for you. It will bring all of your family together. You will feel loved and appreciated like never before

想象一份礼物，我可以向你描述它。这礼物并不大——和高尔夫球差不多大，被包裹成这样。在给你看这礼物之前，我想告诉你，这礼物会对你产生不可思议的影响。这份礼物让你的家人聚在一起，让你感受到关爱并且前所未有地感恩，让你和多年未见的朋友熟人重聚。

and reconnect with friends and acquaintances you haven't heard from in years. Adoration and admiration will overwhelm you. It will recalibrate what's most important in your life.

It will redefine your sense of spirituality and faith. You'll have a new understanding and trust in your body. You'll have unsurpassed vitality and energy. You'll expand your vocabulary, meet new people, and you'll have a healthier lifestyle. And get this—you'll have an eight-week vacation of doing absolutely nothing. You'll eat countless gourmet meals. Flowers will arrive by the truckload. People will say to you, "You look great. Have you had any work done?" And you'll have a lifetime supply of good drugs.

You'll be challenged, inspired, motivated and humbled. Your life will have new meaning. Peace, health, serenity, happiness, nirvana. The price? $55,000, and that's an incredible deal.

By now I know you're dying to know what it is and where you can get one. Does Amazon carry it? Does it have the Apple logo on it? Is there a waiting list? Not likely. This gift came to me about five months ago. It looked more like this when it was all wrapped up—not quite so pretty. And this, and then this. It was a rare gem—a brain tumor,

你心中会充满爱和敬畏。你会重新思考生命中最重要的事情究竟是什么。

这礼物会重新定义你的精神和信仰,你会重新认识和感受自己的身体。你会拥有无穷的生命力和能量。你会有更大的词汇量,认识新的朋友,并且以更健康的方式生活。因为这个礼物,你会有八周的假期,完全不用做任何事。你会享用无尽的美食,成车的鲜花将会送到你的面前。人们会对你说:"你看上去很棒,最近在做什么呢?"你还会得到可以享用一生的良药。

你会接受新的挑战,激发新的灵感,产生新的动力,同时也会更加谦逊。你的人生将会产生新的意义:平和,健康,宁静,幸福,重生。代价是什么呢?五万五千美元,真是一笔划算的买卖。

我想你现在肯定很想知道这礼物是什么,在哪里能买到。亚马逊上能买到吗?礼物上有没有苹果的标志?要排队等货吗?你可能买不到。我是五个月前收到的这份礼物。看上去就像这样,如果包裹起来的话——并不是很好看。看上去是这样的,还有这样的。这份礼物

hemangioblastoma—the gift that keeps on giving.

And while I'm okay now, I wouldn't wish this gift for you. I'm not sure you'd want it. But I wouldn't change my experience. It profoundly altered my life in ways I didn't expect in all the ways I just shared with you.

So the next time you're faced with something that's unexpected, unwanted and uncertain, consider that it just may be a gift.

珍贵而罕见——一颗脑瘤,成血管细胞瘤,一个带给你无尽收获的礼物。

我现在康复了,但我并不希望你也得到这份礼物,我不能确定你是否想要它。但我的经历无可改变,它以意想不到的方式从各个方面改变了我的生活,现在我把这经历与你们共享。

所以下回,当你遇到意外,遇到不想要或是不确定的事,不妨把它看作一份人生的礼物。

Lecture 9   What's So Funny About Mental Illness?

精神病有什么可笑的?

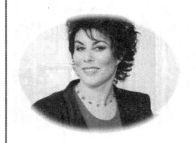

　　卢比·瓦克斯(Ruby Wax)是英国知名的喜剧演员,曾是皇家莎士比亚剧团的一员。她给其他人带来欢笑的同时,却与抑郁症抗争多年。她调侃自己就是那1/4人群中的一员(据世界卫生组织估计,几乎每4人中便有1人会在一生中某个阶段出现精神或行为问题)。她50多岁时考上了牛津大学,学习神经科学和正念认知疗法,并获得牛津大学硕士学位。在学习如何处理自己情绪问题的同时,她成立了一个网站——抑郁患者社团,帮助和支持那些有情绪问题的人们。为表彰卢比·瓦克斯在精神健康领域做出的杰出贡献,2015年英国政府授予她大英帝国勋章。同年,她被聘为塞瑞大学精神健康护理客座教授。

1　One in four people suffer from some sort of mental illness, so if it was one, two, three, four, it's you, sir. You. Yeah. (Laughter) With the weird teeth. And you next to him. (Laughter) You know who you are. Actually, that whole row isn't right. (Laughter) That's not good. Hi. Yeah. Real bad. Don't even look at me. (Laughter)

2　I am one of the one in four. Thank you. I think I inherit it from my mother, who, used to crawl around the house on all fours. She had two *sponges*①in her hand, and then she had two tied to her knees. My mother was completely *absorbent*②. (Laughter) And she would crawl around behind me going, "Who brings footprints into a building?!" So that was kind of a clue that things weren't right. So before I start, I would like to thank the makers of Lamotrigine, Sertraline, and Reboxetine, because without those few simple chemicals, I would not be *vertical*③today.

3　So how did it start? My mental illness—well,

1　每四个人中就有一人患有某种精神疾病,如果让我来数:一、二、三、四,就是你了,先生。对,就是你,牙齿有点怪的那位,还有旁边那位。你知道我说的是谁。事实上那一整排的人都不大正常。这不太好,是的,真的很糟糕。拜托别看着我。

2　其实我就是四个人中的那一位精神病患者,谢谢。我想我是从妈妈那里遗传来的这个毛病,她常常四肢着地在房子里到处爬。她手里拿着两个海绵,还有两个绑在膝盖那里。我妈妈吸水能力超强的(这里是个双关语,absorbent 也可以用来形容人学习能力强)。她会跟在我身后爬来爬去,喊着:"谁把脚印踩进屋子里了?!"从那时的表现你就能看出,她不太正常。所以,在我演讲之前,我想先感谢下拉莫三嗪、舍曲林和帕罗西汀的制药商。因为如果没有这几种常用药物,我今天就不会站在这里了。

3　我的病是怎么开始的呢? 我

---

①　sponge *n.* 海绵,海绵状物
②　absorbent *adj.* 能吸收的
③　vertical *adj.* 垂直的,竖立的

I'm not even going to talk about my mental illness. What am I going to talk about? Okay. I always dreamt that, when I had my final breakdown, it would be because I had a deep Kafkaesque *existentialist*① *revelation*② or that maybe Cate Blanchett would play me and she would win an Oscar for it. But that's not what happened. I had my breakdown during my daughter's sports day. There were all the parents sitting in a parking lot eating food out of the back of their car—only the English—eating their sausages. They loved their sausages. Lord and Lady Rigor Mortis were *nibbling*③ on the *tarmac*④, and then the gun went off and all the girls started running, and all the mommies went, "Run! Run Chlamydia! Run!" "Run like the wind, Veruca! Run!" And all the girls, girls running, running, running, everybody except for my daughter, who was just standing at the starting line, just waving, because she didn't know she was supposed to run. So I took to my bed for about a month, and when I woke up I found I was institutionalized, and when I saw the other *inmates*⑤, I realized that I had found my people, my tribe. Because they became my only friends, they became my friends, because very

根本不想谈论我的精神疾病。可我还能谈些什么呢? 好吧。我常常会想,我发病的诱因,要么是深受卡夫卡式存在主义的启示,要么是因为凯特·布兰切特扮演了我的角色并赢得了奥斯卡奖。但这些都没有发生。我发病的时候,正是我女儿的运动会。所有家长都坐在停车场,吃着后备厢里带的食物——全是英国人——他们吃着香肠,他们可喜欢香肠了。僵尸爵爷和夫人正在柏油马路上啃食,突然间枪声响了,所有的女孩都跑了起来,所有的妈妈都喊着:"快跑! 快跑,克莱米迪亚! 快跑!""像风一样跑,维鲁卡! 快跑!"(演讲者在这里特意用了两个与病谐音的姓名:chlamydia 为衣原体,verruca 为疣)所有的女孩都在跑啊跑,除了我的女儿。她就站在起跑线那儿,光顾着挥手,因为她不知道她应该跑起来。我因此卧床一个月,醒来的时候,已经住进了精神病院。看到其他病人,我意识到自己找到了组织。他们成了我唯一的朋友,因为我认识的人都没

---

① existentialist *n.* 存在主义者
② revelation *n.* 启示
③ nibble *v.* 啃,一点一点地咬
④ tarmac *n.* 柏油路面
⑤ inmate *n.* 室友,尤指同院病人

few people that I knew—Well, I wasn't sent a lot of cards or flowers. I mean, if I had had a broken leg or I was with child, I would have been *inundated*①, but all I got was a couple phone calls telling me to *perk up*②. Perk up. Because I didn't think of that. (Laughter)

4　Because, you know, the one thing, one thing that you get with this disease, this one comes with a package, is you get a real sense of shame, because your friends go, "Oh come on, show me the *lump*③, show me the X-rays," and of course you've got nothing to show, so you're, like, really disgusted with yourself because you're thinking, "I'm not being carpet-bombed. I don't live in a township." So you start to hear these abusive voices, but you don't hear one abusive voice, you hear about a thousand—100,000 abusive voices, like if the Devil had *Tourette's*④, that's what it would sound like. But we all know in here, you know, there is no Devil, there are no voices in your head. You know that when you have those abusive voices, all those little neurons get together and in that little gap you get a real *toxic*⑤"I want to kill myself" kind of chemical,

有来看我——嗯,我并没有收到很多慰问卡片或花束。我的意思是,如果我摔断了腿,或者我生孩子了,或许会被鲜花和问候卡淹没了。但那时我只接到了几通电话叫我振作。好吧,振作。可能我以前都不知道要振作吧。

4　得了这种病,随之而来的还有一种很丢脸的感觉。一般生病的时候,你的朋友会说:"来,给我看看肿块,给我看看 X 光片。"可是得了这种病,你却没什么能拿来展示的。你会厌恶自己,因为你觉得"没有那么多人来探视,我都不像是生活在城里的人。"你开始听到很多谩骂声,不是一声两声,而是成千上万的谩骂声,就像恶魔患了多动秽语综合征一样,是的,听起来就像那样。但在座的各位都知道,并没有恶魔,你的头脑中并没有声音。当你听到那些谩骂声的时候,你脑袋里面那些小神经元都挤进了一个小狭缝,使你的脑中产生一种有毒物质,让你不断产生自杀的念头。如果这种情况一再出现,你可能

---

①　inundate *v.* 泛滥,淹没
②　perk up 振作
③　lump *n.* 肿块
④　Tourette's *n.* 秽语综合征
⑤　toxic *n.* 毒物,毒剂

and if you have that over and over again on a *loop tape*①, you might have yourself depression. Oh, and that's not even the tip of the iceberg. If you get a little baby, and you abuse it verbally, its little brain sends out chemicals that are so destructive that the little part of its brain that can tell good from bad just doesn't grow, so you might have yourself a homegrown *psychotic*②. If a soldier sees his friend blown up, his brain goes into such high alarm that he can't actually put the experience into words, so he just feels the horror over and over again.

就会陷入抑郁。哦，这些连冰山一角都算不上。如果你对家里的孩子使用这种语言暴力，他的小脑袋里产生的化学物质，甚至会破坏他分辨善恶的能力，一个精神病患者就这样养成了。你可以把精神病患者想象成一个目睹朋友被炸飞的士兵，他的大脑会进入高度戒备的状态，他甚至无法把自己的经历用语言表达出来，只能一直处于恐惧的折磨中。

5 So here's my question. My question is, how come when people have mental damage, it's always an active imagination? How come every other organ in your body can get sick and you get sympathy, except the brain?

5 我于是就有了一个疑问，那就是，为什么人们在遭受精神创伤的时候，总会有活跃的想象力？为什么身体其他器官生病时，你会得到慰问，而大脑生病了却得不到呢？

6 I'd like to talk a little bit more about the brain, because I know you like that here at TED, so if you just give me a minute here, okay. Okay, let me just say, there's some good news. There is some good news. First of all, let me say, we've come a long, long way. We

6 我再来谈谈大脑吧。我知道，来 TED 的听众大都喜欢这个话题。请给我一点时间好吗？这么说吧，我有好消息。首先，我想说，这是一段非常非常漫长的进化旅程。我们从超级超级小的单细胞变形虫，小到只能贴在石

---

① loop tape 循环磁带
② psychotic *n.* 精神病患者

started off as a teeny, teeny little one-celled *amoeba*①, tiny, just sticking onto a rock, and now, voila, the brain. Here we go. This little baby has a lot of horsepower. It comes completely conscious. It's got state-of-the-art *lobes*②. We've got the *occipital lobe*③ so we can actually see the world. We got the *temporal lobe*④ so we can actually hear the world. Here we've got a little bit of long-term memory, so, you know that night you want to forget, when you got really drunk? Bye-bye! Gone. (Laughter) So actually, it's filled with 100 billion neurons just zizzing away, electrically transmitting information, zizzing, zizzing. I'm going to give you a little side view here. I don't know if you can get that here. So, zizzing away, and so—And for everyone—I know, I drew this myself. Thank you. For every one single neuron, you can actually have from 10,000 to 100,000 different connections or *dendrites*⑤ or whatever you want to call it, and every time you learn something, or you have an experience, that bush grows, you know, that bush of information. Can you imagine, every human being is carrying that equipment, even Paris Hilton? (Laughter) Go figure.

头上的那种,到现在,瞧,进化出了一颗脑袋。就是它了。这颗小脑袋瓜子马力十足,有着完全意识,也有着最先进的脑叶。因为有枕叶,我们能看到世界;因为有颞叶,我们能听到世界上的声音。这是我们储存长期记忆的部分。你很想忘记那个丢脸的醉酒的晚上?拜拜,记忆消失啦!事实上,大脑有 1 000 亿个神经元,嗞嗞,嗞嗞,它们传导着信息,嗞嗞,嗞嗞。我再给你们看一个侧视图。我不知道你们能不能看清楚。对!这是我自己画的。谢谢!事实上每一个神经元都有 1 万到 10 万个连接,或者叫神经树突。但不管你叫它什么,每当你学新东西或有新的经历的时候,这些信息的"树突"就会长大一些。你可以想象么?每个人都有那样的装备,甚至是帕丽斯·希尔顿(全美最出名的希尔顿家族继承人,被称为含着钻石汤匙出生的人,曾因炫富及各种绯闻事件成为大众关注焦点)。想想吧。

---

① amoeba *n.* 变形虫
② lobe *n.* 脑叶
③ occipital lobe 枕叶
④ temporal lobe 颞叶
⑤ dendrite *n.* 树突

7 But I got a little bad news for you folks. I got some bad news. This isn't for the one in four. This is for the four in four. We are not equipped for the 21st century. Evolution did not prepare us for this. We just don't have the *bandwidth*①, and for people who say, oh, they're having a nice day, they're perfectly fine, they're more insane than the rest of us. Because I'll show you where there might be a few *glitches*②in evolution. Okay, let me just explain this to you. When we were ancient man—millions of years ago, and we suddenly felt threatened by a *predator*③, okay? —we would, thank you. I drew these myself. (Laughter) Thank you very much. Thank you. Thank you. Thank you. Anyway, we would fill up with our own *adrenaline*④and our own *cortisol*⑤, and then we'd kill or be killed, we'd eat or we'd be eaten, and then suddenly we'd *defuel*⑥, and we'd go back to normal. Okay. So the problem is, nowadays, with modern man—when we feel in danger, we still fill up with our own chemical but because we can't kill *traffic wardens*⑦—or eat *estate agents*⑧, the fuel just stays in our body over and over, so we're in

7 不过我这里也有坏消息。这不仅是针对那1/4人群的,而是针对每一个人的坏消息。我们的装备还没有准备好进入21世纪,我们还没有进化好。我们的带宽不够。那些说着"哦,我这一天过得棒极了",或者说自己很好的人,其实他们比所有人都不正常。我会把进化过程中的一些小差错展示给你们看。好,让我解释给你们听。几百万年以前,当我们还是古人的时候,我们突然受到掠食动物的威胁——谢谢啊,这是我自己画的,非常感谢——这个时候,我们的肾上腺素和皮质醇会飙升。然后我们要么杀了那些动物,要么被杀;要么把那些动物吃了,要么被吃。等激素水平下降后,我们就回归正常了。很好。但问题来了,作为现代人,当我们感到危险时,我们体内的激素也会飙升,但由于我们不能杀掉交通警察或是吃掉房产中介,这些像燃料一样的激素就一直在体内积攒,所以我们会长期处于

---

① bandwidth *n.* 带宽
② glitch *n.* 小过失,小过错
③ predator *n.* 食肉动物
④ adrenaline *n.* 肾上腺素
⑤ cortisol *n.* 皮质醇
⑥ defuel *v.* 放油,排油
⑦ traffic warden 交通管制员
⑧ estate agent 房地产经纪人

a constant state of alarm, a constant state. And here's another thing that happened. About 150,000 years ago, when language came online, we started to put words to this constant emergency, so it wasn't just, "Oh my God, there's a saber-toothed tiger," which could be, it was suddenly, "Oh my God, I didn't send the email. Oh my God, my thighs are too fat. Oh my God, everybody can see I'm stupid. I didn't get invited to the Christmas party!" So you've got this nagging loop tape that goes over and over again that drives you insane, so, you see what the problem is? What once made you safe now drives you insane. I'm sorry to be the bearer of bad news, but somebody has to be. Your pets are happier than you are. (Laughter) So kitty cat, meow, happy, happy, happy, human beings, screwed. Completely and utterly—so, screwed.

8   But my point is, if we don't talk about this stuff, and we don't learn how to deal with our lives, it's not going to be one in four. It's going to be four in four who are really, really going to get ill in the upstairs department. And while we're at it, can we please stop the *stigma*.① Thank you. (Applause)

9   Thank you.

———————————

① stigma *n.* 耻辱,污名

高警戒状态中,这成为常态。还有件事儿也值得一提。大概15万年前,我们开始使用语言。我们会用语言来描述这些经常发生的紧急事件。这些语言从曾经的"天啊,那儿有只剑齿虎"突然变成了"天啊,我没发邮件! 天啊! 我的大腿好粗! 天啊! 大家都在看我笑话了! 天啊! 圣诞派对居然没邀请我!"这些烦人的声音一次次被重播,快把你逼疯了。好了,你看到问题的症结了吧? 曾经让你感到安全的东西,现在正把你逼疯。我很抱歉成为坏消息的传递者,但总得有人做这事。事实上你的宠物比你更快乐。小猫咪,喵,快乐又开心。人类,完蛋了! 彻底完蛋了!

8   我其实想说的是,如果我们对这件事避而不谈,如果我们不学着应对我们的生活中的压力,那就真的不仅是四分之一,而是所有的人都得到精神科就诊了。要真是那样的话,我们可不可以不再给精神问题冠以污名?

9   谢谢!

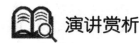 演讲赏析

这是一篇有关价值问题的说服性演讲（persuasive speech on questions of values）。演讲者以"问题—成因—出路"（problem-cause-solution）的顺序展开论证，说服听众摒弃对精神病患者的偏见，鼓励所有深受情绪问题折磨的人们，笑对人生的考验。

演讲者开头通过单项数据（single statistic）——每四个人里就有一个人精神上有毛病，达到了震撼听众（startle the audience）的效果。随后关联听众（relate to the audience），与听众建立了良好的关系（create a positive relationship with the audience），有效地激起了听众继续听下去的兴趣（get the attention and interest of your audience）。

文章的主体分为两个部分。首先演讲者描述了自己的亲身经历（personal experience），作为精神病患者的女儿，她遗传了母亲的精神疾病。而在女儿的运动会上，她自己的精神病发作了。患病后的经历让演讲者开始思考，与其他疾病患者相比，为什么精神病患者得不到别人的同情？这是向听众提出的问题（problem），也是演讲者的第一个论点（main point one）。演讲者自身形象生动的故事（extended examples），很容易把听众带进演讲里，同时建立了自己的可信度（credibility）。在第二部分，演讲者分析了精神问题的原因——大脑还没对 21 世纪做好准备（main point two），说服听众同情精神病患者。演讲者在解释人类大脑时借助了大脑模型（model）和图画（drawings）的视觉辅助手段（visual aids），生动有趣，帮助听众很好地理解了大脑的结构和运作。在解释为什么有些人大脑会持续处于警戒状态时，演讲者运用了类比论证（analogical reasoning）的方法：古代人可以通过杀戮瞬间让有害情绪得到释放，而在现代社会，人们只能通过语言来释放压力，而不断地抱怨会产生情绪问题。演讲者用生动活泼的语言代替了枯燥难懂的行话（jargon），有效地向听众传达了信息。

文章结尾部分，演讲者提出了解决方法（solution），希望听众处理好自己的生活，同时不再给精神病患者冠以污名。

本篇演讲最大的特点是：演讲者肢体动作丰富，语言风趣幽默、富有感染力。作为精神问题的受害者，她将论证融于情感之中（appealing to emotions），其自信乐观的精神面貌鼓励和劝服了听众。

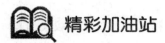

精彩加油站

精彩视频

Programming Bacteria to Detect Cancer
（and Maybe Treat it）
利用细菌发现癌症(也许还能治愈它)

You may not realize this, but there are more bacteria in your body than stars in our entire galaxy. This fascinating universe of bacteria inside of us is an integral part of our health, and our technology is evolving so rapidly that today we can program these bacteria like we program computers.

Now, the diagram that you see here, I know it looks like some kind of sports play, but it is actually a blueprint of the first bacterial program I developed. And like writing software, we can print and write DNA into different algorithms and programs inside of bacteria. What this program does is produce fluorescent proteins in a rhythmic fashion and generate a small molecule that allows bacteria to communicate and synchronize, as you're seeing in this movie. The growing colony of bacteria that you see here is about the width of a human hair. Now, what you can't see is that our genetic program instructs these bacteria to each produce small molecules, and these molecules

或许你并没有意识到,你身体里的细菌比银河系中的星星还要多。我们体内这迷人的"细菌宇宙"是我们身体健康不可缺少的部分,而科技的迅速发展让我们可以像处理计算机程序一样处理这些细菌。

现在你看到的这张图,看起来有点像是某种体育运动的示意图,但实际上它是我开发的第一个细菌程序。就像写软件代码那样,我们可以根据不同的算法输出和撰写 DNA 序列,并在细菌内部编写程序。这个程序做的事情,正如你在这个影片里所看到的,就是按照一定的节奏制造荧光蛋白,并生成小分子,让细菌可以彼此联系,实现信息同步。这个成长中的菌落,大小和人类头发的宽度差不多。但你们看不到的是,我们的基因程序正在指导这些细菌各自产生小分子。这些分子在数千个细菌个体之间游移,通知它们什么时候开启和关闭

travel between the thousands of individual bacteria telling them when to turn on and off. And the bacteria synchronize quite well at this scale, but because the molecule that synchronizes them together can only travel so fast, in larger colonies of bacteria, this results in traveling waves between bacteria that are far away from each other, and you can see these waves going from right to left across the screen.

Now, our genetic program relies on a natural phenomenon called quorum sensing, in which bacteria trigger coordinated and sometimes virulent behaviors once they reach a critical density. You can observe quorum sensing in action in this movie, where a growing colony of bacteria only begins to glow once it reaches a high or critical density. Our genetic program continues producing these rhythmic patterns of fluorescent proteins as the colony grows outwards. This particular movie and experiment we call The Supernova, because it looks like an exploding star.

Now, besides programming these beautiful patterns, I wondered, what else can we get these bacteria to do? And I decided to explore how we can program bacteria to detect and treat diseases in our bodies like cancer. One of the surprising facts about bacteria is that they can naturally grow inside

相应的功能。在这个范围内，细菌同步表现得很好。但在比较大的菌落里，这些让细菌同步的分子的快速移动，会导致相距较远的细菌个体间产生传导波动。你们可以在荧幕上看到这种波动，从右向左移动。

我们的基因程序依赖于一种叫做"群体感应"的自然现象：一旦菌落达到临界密度，细菌之间就会激发相互协调甚至致命的行为。在这段视频中，你能观察到活动中的"群体感应"现象。只有达到高密度或临界密度的时候，成长中的菌落才会开始发光。在菌落向外成长蔓延时，我们的基因程序会持续有节奏地制造荧光蛋白。我们称这段特别的影像和实验为"超级新星"，因为看起来很像恒星大爆炸。

我开始思考，除了编译这些美丽的图样外，我们还能让这些细菌做什么？我决定探索如何对细菌进行编程，从而发现和治疗体内疾病，如癌症。细菌的一个惊人之处在于，它们可以在肿瘤内部自然地生长。这是因为，免疫系统通常影响

of tumors. This happens because typically tumors are areas where the immune system has no access, and so bacteria find these tumors and use them as a safe haven to grow and thrive. We started using probiotic bacteria which are safe bacteria that have a health benefit, and found that when orally delivered to mice, these probiotics would selectively grow inside of liver tumors. We realized that the most convenient way to highlight the presence of the probiotics, and hence, the presence of the tumors, was to get these bacteria to produce a signal that would be detectable in the urine, and so we specifically programmed these probiotics to make a molecule that would change the color of your urine to indicate the presence of cancer. We went on to show that this technology could sensitively and specifically detect liver cancer, one that is challenging to detect otherwise.

Now, since these bacteria specifically localize to tumors, we've been programming them to not only detect cancer but also to treat cancer by producing therapeutic molecules from within the tumor environment that shrink the existing tumors, and we've been doing this using quorum sensing programs like you saw in the previous movies.

Altogether, imagine in the future, taking

不到肿瘤,所以当细菌发现这些肿瘤时,会将肿瘤当作避风港,在里面茁壮成长。我们开始使用益生菌,它们安全并对健康有益。后来发现,当老鼠口服益生菌时,这些益生菌会选择生长在肝脏肿瘤里。我们意识到,为了方便标记出益生菌,从而追踪到肿瘤,可以让这些益生菌产生一种在尿液中能检测到的信号。因此我们特别编译了这些益生菌,让它们产生能改变尿液颜色的分子,从而实现癌症的检测。我们随后证明了这项技术在肝癌检测中的高灵敏度和准确度,而通过其他方式是很难检测到肝癌的。

既然这些细菌能准确定位肿瘤,我们又试着对细菌进行编译,让它们不仅能检测癌症,还能治疗癌症。我们让肿瘤内部产生治疗分子,让现有的肿瘤萎缩。就像你们在之前的视频中看到的一样,我们已经用群体感应程序来实现这一过程了。

总之,想象一下,将来通过服用

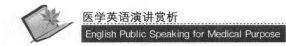

a programmed probiotic that could detect and treat cancer, or even other diseases. Our ability to program bacteria and program life opens up new horizons in cancer research, and to share this vision, I worked with artist Vik Muniz to create the symbol of the universe, made entirely out of bacteria or cancer cells. Ultimately, my hope is that the beauty and purpose of this microscopic universe can inspire new and creative approaches for the future of cancer research.

Thank you.

这些被编译过的细菌,我们可以检测和治疗癌症以及其他疾病。我们能对细菌和生命进行编程,为癌症研究打开新的视野。为了分享这个美好的愿景,我和艺术家维克·穆尼斯合作,创作了这个完全由细菌和癌症细胞组成的宇宙符号。最后,我希望这个美丽的微观世界,有其存在的意义,它能在未来激发出创新的癌症研究方法。

谢谢。

Lecture 10   The Mystery of Chronic Pain
慢性疼痛之谜

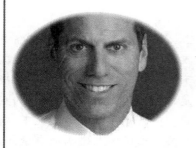

艾略特·克莱恩（Elliot Krane）毕业于美国亚利桑那大学医学院，是美国斯坦福大学露西尔·帕卡德儿童医院的一位儿科医生，拥有美国麻醉师资格评定委员会的认证及美国儿科委员会的认证。他是医院疼痛管理服务中心的负责人，长期致力于帮助青少年儿童解决慢性疼痛问题，擅长研究和治疗进行了手术的儿童、患有糖尿病并发症的儿童，以及由于神经损伤而饱受神经性疼痛困扰的儿童。

1   I'm a pediatrician and an ***anesthesiologist***①, so I put children to sleep for a living. (Laughter) And I'm an academic, so I put audiences to sleep for free. (Laughter) But what I actually mostly do is I manage the pain management service at the Packard Children's Hospital up at Stanford in Palo Alto. And it's from the experience from about 20 or 25 years of doing that that I want to bring to you the message this morning, that pain is a disease.

2   Now most of the time, you think of pain as a symptom of a disease, and that's true most of the time. It's the symptom of a ***tumor***②or an infection or an ***inflammation***③or an operation. But about 10 percent of the time, after the patient has recovered from one of those events, pain persists. It persists for months and often times for years, and when that happens, it is its own disease. And before I tell you about how it is that we think that happens and what we can do about it, I want to show you how it feels for my patients. So imagine, if you will, that I'm stroking your arm with this feather, as I'm stroking my arm right now. Now, I want you to imagine that I'm stroking it with this. Please keep your seat. (Laughter) A very different feeling. Now what does it have to do with

1   我是一名儿科医生,同时还是一名麻醉师,我的工作是让孩子们睡着。(笑声)我也是一名大学教师,所以我可以免费让听我课的人睡着。(笑声)但我的主要工作是在帕罗奥多市斯坦福大学的帕卡德儿童医院提供疼痛管理服务。根据我20或25年的执业经验,今早,我想告诉你的是,疼痛是一种病。

2   很多时候,你会认为疼痛是疾病的一种症状。在大多数情况下,这种想法是正确的。它的确是肿瘤、感染、发炎或手术后的症状。但仍有约10%的情况下,病人虽然已经从上述病况中康复,但疼痛仍然持续。有时持续数月,有时甚至持续数年。当这种情况发生时,疼痛本身就是一种疾病。在我告诉你它是如何发生的以及我们可以采取何种措施之前,我想向你们展示一下病人对疼痛的感受。如果可以,请你想象一下,我用这根羽毛挠你,就像现在我挠自己的手臂一样。现在,再请你想象一下,如果我用这个东西(喷火枪)"挠"你呢?请坐

---

①   anesthesiologist *n.* 麻醉师

②   tumor *n.* 肿瘤

③   inflammation *n.* 感染

chronic pain? Imagine, if you will, these two ideas together. Imagine what your life would be like if I were to stroke it with this feather, but your brain was telling you that this is what you are feeling—and that is the experience of my patients with chronic pain. In fact, imagine something even worse. Imagine I were to stroke your child's arm with this feather, and their brain [was] telling them that they were feeling this hot torch.

好！（笑声）完全不同的感觉。这跟慢性疼痛有什么关系呢？如果可以的话，请想象一下，将这两种感觉混合在一起。如果我用这根羽毛去挠你，但你的大脑却告诉你，这是灼伤的感觉，那么，你的生活将会变成怎样？——这就是我的患者对慢性疼痛的感受。事实上，想象一下更糟糕的情况。想象一下我用这根羽毛去挠你孩子的胳膊，但他们的大脑却告诉他们，他们感受到的是这个灼热的喷火枪。

3　That was the experience of my patient, Chandler, whom you see in the photograph. As you can see, she's a beautiful, young woman. She was 16 years old last year when I met her, and she aspired to be a professional dancer. And during the course of one of her dance rehearsals, she fell on her *outstretched*①arm and *sprained*②her wrist. Now you would probably imagine, as she did, that a *wrist*③sprain is a trivial event in a person's life. Wrap it in an ACE *bandage*④, take some *ibuprofen*⑤for a week or two, and that's the end of the story. But in Chandler's case, that

3　这就是我的患者钱德勒的遭遇，就是照片中的这个女孩。正如你看到的，她是个漂亮又年轻的姑娘。去年我遇到她时，她16岁，渴望成为一名专业的舞者。在一次舞蹈排练过程中，她摔到了自己向外伸展的手臂，并且扭伤了手腕。你可能跟她想的一样，认为这是人生中再普通不过的一次受伤。用布织绷带缠起来，吃一到两周的布洛芬，这件事就这么过去了。但是在钱德勒的这次遭遇中，这只是故事的开始。

---

①　outstretched *adj.* 伸展的
②　sprain *v.* 扭伤
③　wrist *n.* 手腕
④　bandage *n.* 绷带
⑤　ibuprofen *n.* 布洛芬,异丁苯丙酸

was the beginning of the story. This is what her arm looked like when she came to my clinic about three months after her sprain. You can see that the arm is **discolored**①, purplish in color. It was **cadaverically**② cold to the touch. The muscles were frozen, **paralyzed**③—**dystonic**④ is how we refer to that. The pain had spread from her wrist to her hands, to her fingertips, from her wrist up to her elbow, almost all the way to her shoulder.

4　But the worst part was, not the **spontaneous**⑤ pain that was there 24 hours a day. The worst part was that she had **allodynia**⑥, the medical term for the phenomenon that I just illustrated with the feather and with the torch. The lightest touch of her arm—the touch of a hand, the touch even of a sleeve, of a garment, as she put it on—caused **excruciating**⑦, burning pain.

5　How can the nervous system get this so wrong? How can the nervous system

图中是她来我诊所时，手臂的样子，这已经是扭伤发生约三个月后了。你可以看到她的手臂已经变色，有点发紫，摸上去像尸体一样冷。肌肉僵硬、麻痹，就是我们常说的肌张力异常。疼痛从她的手腕蔓延到手掌、到手指，又从手腕蔓延到手肘，直到她的肩膀。

4　但最糟糕的不是每天24小时的自发性疼痛。最糟糕的是她患上了痛觉超敏症。这是一个医学术语，说的就是我刚才用羽毛和喷火枪所演示的那种情况。轻微地触碰她的手臂——比如别人手掌的触碰，甚至只是她自己穿衣时碰到了袖子或者衣服——都会造成难以忍受的烧灼痛。

5　神经系统怎么会犯这样的错呢？怎么会把像手的触摸那样无

---

① discolored *adj.* 变色的

② cadaverically *adv.* 尸体的

③ paralyzed *adj.* 瘫痪的，麻痹的

④ dystonic *adj.* 张力障碍的

⑤ spontaneous *adj.* 自发的

⑥ allodynia *n.* 异常性疼痛

⑦ excruciating *adj.* 极度的，剧痛的

misinterpret an innocent *sensation*①like the touch of a hand and turn it into the *malevolent*②sensation of the touch of the flame? Well you probably imagine that the nervous system in the body is hardwired like your house. In your house, wires run in the wall, from the light switch to a junction box in the ceiling and from the junction box to the light bulb. And when you turn the switch on, the light goes on. And when you turn the switch off, the light goes off. So people imagine the nervous system is just like that. If you hit your thumb with a hammer, these wires in your arm—that, of course, we call nerves—transmit the information into the junction box in the spinal cord where new wires, new nerves, take the information up to the brain where you become consciously aware that your thumb is now hurt.

6　But the situation, of course, in the human body is far more complicated than that. Instead of it being the case that that junction box in the *spinal cord*③is just simple where one nerve connects with the next nerve by releasing these little brown packets of chemical information called *neurotransmitters*④in a *linear*⑤one-on-

害的感觉误解为一个像火焰灼烧那样伤害性的感觉呢？嗯，也许你可以把身体里的神经系统想象成家里的电线电路。在你家里，电线穿过墙壁，把灯的开关与天花板上的接线盒、接线盒与灯泡连接起来。当你打开开关的时候，灯泡亮了。当你关闭开关的时候，灯泡熄灭。所以人们认为神经系统就是这样工作的。如果你用锤子砸到了大拇指，你手臂里的电线——当然，这里我们应该称之为神经——在脊髓里传递信息到接线盒。通过接线盒，新电线，即新的神经，把信息运送到大脑，因此你能意识到你的大拇指受伤了。

6　当然，身体里的情况，实际上要复杂得多。在位于脊髓的这个接线盒里，神经和神经联结的方式并不是一对一的线性方式，即通过单向释放这种携带化学信息的棕色小块——神经递质——来联结。事实上，神经递质在脊髓

---

① sensation *n.* 感觉，知觉
② malevolent *adj.* 恶毒的
③ spinal cord *n.* 脊髓
④ neurotransmitter *n.* 神经传递素
⑤ linear *adj.* 线性的

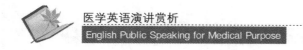
one fashion, in fact, what happens is the neurotransmitters spill out in three dimensions—*laterally*①, *vertically*②, up and down in the spinal cord—and they start interacting with other *adjacent*③ cells. These cells, called *glial cells*④, were once thought to be unimportant structural elements of the spinal cord that did nothing more than hold all the important things together, like the nerves. But it turns out the glial cells have a vital role in the *modulation*⑤, *amplification*⑥ and, in the case of pain, the *distortion*⑦ of sensory experiences. These glial cells become activated. Their DNA starts to *synthesize*⑧ new proteins, which spill out and interact with adjacent nerves, and they start releasing their neurotransmitters, and those neurotransmitters spill out and activate adjacent glial cells, and so on and so forth, until what we have is a positive feedback loop.

7　It's almost as if somebody came into your home and rewired your walls so that the next time you turned on the light switch, the toilet flushed three doors down, or your dishwasher

里的传递方向是三个维度的——横向、纵向和上下，它也会和邻近的细胞发生反应。这些细胞，被称为神经胶质细胞，曾经被认为是脊髓里不重要的结构组成，它们的作用仅仅是用来支撑类似于神经这样的重要结构。可是后来才发现，神经胶质细胞在调节、扩大、歪曲（在疼痛案例中）感觉体验的过程中起着非常重要的作用。这些胶质细胞被激活，它们的 DNA 开始合成新的蛋白质，这些蛋白质扩散并与邻近的神经发生反应，然后释放出神经递质。这些神经递质又被释放出来，激活了邻近的胶质细胞。如此循环往复，直到形成了一个正反馈循环。

7　这就好像有人去了你家，重新在你家墙壁里布线。结果你下次打开灯的开关，却意外地冲了三次马桶，或是启动了洗碗机，或

---

①　laterally *adv.* 侧面地，横向地
②　vertically *adv.* 垂直地
③　adjacent *adj.* 临近的
④　glial cell *n.* 神经胶质细胞
⑤　modulation *n.* 调节
⑥　amplification *n.* 扩大
⑦　distortion *n.* 扭曲，变形
⑧　synthesize *v.* 合成

went on, or your computer monitor turned off. That's crazy, but that's, in fact, what happens with chronic pain. And that's why pain becomes its own disease. The nervous system has *plasticity*①. It changes, and it *morphs*②in response to stimuli.

8   Well, what do we do about that? What can we do in a case like Chandler's? We treat these patients in a rather crude fashion at this point in time. We treat them with symptom-modifying drugs—painkillers—which are, frankly, not very effective for this kind of pain. We take nerves that are noisy and active that should be quiet, and we put them to sleep with local *anesthetics*③. And most importantly, what we do is we use a rigorous, and often uncomfortable, process of physical therapy and occupational therapy to retrain the nerves in the nervous system to respond normally to the activities and sensory experiences that are part of everyday life. And we support all of that with an intensive *psychotherapy*④program to address the *despondency*⑤, despair and depression that always accompanies severe, chronic pain.

是关闭了电脑显示器。这很不可思议,但事实上,这就是患上慢性疼痛后会发生的事情。这也解释了为什么疼痛本身会变成一种疾病。神经系统有可塑性。面对刺激,它会改变,也会变异。

8   我们该怎么办呢?在像钱德勒这样的案例中我们该如何去做呢?我们目前采用的治疗方法还不是很完善。我们用缓解症状的药物——止疼药——来治疗病患,坦白说,对于这种疼痛并不是很有效。我们也用局部麻醉的方法,让那些过度活跃的神经进入休眠。最重要的是,我们还会采用严格的,但往往令人不太舒服的物理疗法和作业疗法来修正神经应答,使它们在日常的活动和感官体验中能做出正常的反应。另外,我们还会用集中心理治疗配合上述治疗,以解决那些伴随着严重慢性疼痛而来的沮丧、绝望和抑郁问题。

---

① plasticity *n.* 黏性,可塑性
② morph *v.* 变种,改变
③ anesthetics *n.* 麻醉剂
④ psychotherapy *n.* 心理治疗
⑤ despondency *n.* 沮丧,失望

9   It's successful, as you can see from this video of Chandler, who, two months after we first met her, is now doing a back flip. And I had lunch with her yesterday because she's a college student studying dance at Long Beach here, and she's doing absolutely fantastic.

10   But the future is actually even brighter. The future holds the promise that new drugs will be developed that are not symptom-modifying drugs that simply mask the problem, as we have now, but that will be disease-modifying drugs that will actually go right to the root of the problem and attack those glial cells, or those *pernicious*①proteins that the glial cells elaborate, that spill over and cause this central nervous system wind-up, or plasticity, that so is capable of distorting and amplifying the sensory experience that we call pain. So I have hoped that in the future, the prophetic words of George Carlin will be realized, who said, "My philosophy: No pain, no pain."

11   Thank you very much.

9   我们成功了。正如你在这个视频中看到的,在我们见面两个月后,钱德勒可以做后空翻了。昨天我刚和她一起吃了午饭,她正在长滩这里的大学学习舞蹈。她简直是棒极了。

10   未来会更加美好。我们将有希望开发新的药物。和我们现在用的那些仅能粉饰问题、缓解症状的药物不同,新的药物可以治疗疾病,真正从根本上解决问题。它们可以针对神经胶质细胞起作用,也可以针对由神经胶质细胞产生并溢出的有害蛋白质起作用(这种溢出往往会造成中枢神经系统紊乱),还可以针对神经系统的可塑性起作用(该可塑性会歪曲并放大我们的疼痛感受)。所以,我有一个愿望。将来,乔治·卡林的预言会实现,即:"我的哲学是:没有疼痛就不会疼痛。"

11   非常感谢。

---

①   pernicious *adj.* 有害的,恶性的

演讲赏析

这是一篇成功的说解性演讲(informative speech)。演讲者采用时间顺序法(chronological order)描述了患者钱德勒的遭遇以及对她病况的处置方法,清晰而又生动地解释了慢性疼痛这一概念。

在演讲的开头部分,演讲者以幽默的语言引起听众的注意(get attention and interest),并直截了当地点明了演讲的主题:疼痛是一种病。

在演讲的主体部分,演讲者首先使用了羽毛和喷火枪这两种道具(objects and models),并让听众想象(hypothetical examples)当这二者触碰身体后,正常人和病患者不同的疼痛体验,使听众对慢性疼痛这种疾病有了更深的了解,同时引发了听众的好奇感(arouse curiosity)。其次,演讲者描述了患者钱德勒的遭遇和病情,并使用了打比方的修辞手法(simile and metaphor),将人体的神经系统比喻成家庭的电路电线,避免了过于学术化的描述,使听众明白了慢性疼痛发生的原理。接下来,演讲者介绍了医生们对患者钱德勒所采取的治疗措施,并通过视频(video)这一视觉辅助手段(visual aids),告知听众钱德勒的治疗结果,证明了治疗方法的有效性。

在演讲的最后,演讲者回顾并总结了(reinforce the central idea and summarize your speech)造成慢性疼痛的主要原因:1. *those glial cells*;2. *those pernicious proteins that the glial cells elaborate, that spill over and cause this central nervous system wind-up*;3. *plasticity that so is capable of distorting and amplifying the sensory experience*,并在此基础上提出了对新药研发工作的展望。最后,演讲者引用了(end with a quotation)美国演员乔治·卡林的话:没有疼痛就不会疼痛,将演讲主题完美的升华。

纵观整个演讲,演讲者的语言幽默诙谐,肢体动作(gestures and movements)得体大方,图片(photographs and drawings)、视频(video)、道具(objects and models)等多个视觉辅助手段(visual aids)使用恰当。考虑到听众的实际水平,演讲者尽可能地减少了行话(jargon)和术语(technical terms)的使用,条理清晰地为听众解开了慢性疼痛之谜。

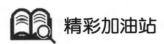 精彩加油站

Peng Liyuan's Speech in Geneva
彭丽媛在瑞士日内瓦出席亲善大使任期续延暨颁奖仪式上的致辞

精彩视频

Director-General Margaret Chan, Executive Director Michelle Sidibe,

It's a great honor to be back. I am deeply humbled by your kind words.

Dr. Chan and Mr. Sidibe, you are the real champions in the fight to end killer disease and keep our world healthy and safe. It's been a privilege to work with you and everyone else in this room.

Standing here five and a half years ago, when WHO named me Goodwill Ambassador, I said, "I hope to contribute to the great work of WHO in saving lives from TB and HIV/AIDS, and help those most at risk." Before that, I had been China's ambassador for HIV/AIDS for five years and TB for four years, so I knew what we were up against and what would happen if we did not work hard or act fast enough.

尊敬的陈冯富珍总干事,尊敬的西迪贝执行主任:

很荣幸能再次来到世界卫生组织总部。感谢你们热情洋溢的致辞。

陈冯富珍总干事和西迪贝执行主任,你们在全球抗击致命疾病和促进人类健康与安全方面发挥着极其重要的领导作用。我很高兴能够和你们以及在座的各位一起为这一事业而努力。

五年半前,同样在这里,世界卫生组织任命我为结核病和艾滋病防治亲善大使。在任命仪式上,我表示:"我希望为世卫组织救治结核病和艾滋病患者的伟大事业尽一份力,并帮助那些高危人群。"在那之前,我在中国已分别担任了五年时间的预防艾滋病宣传员和四年时间的防治结核病宣传形象大使。因此,我十分了解全球在抗击结核病与艾滋病方面所面临的挑战,也非

Since 2006，I have been to high-risk places, villages, hospitals, patients' homes, community centers, schools and universities and research centers to understand the challenge and call for action. I have seen pain and fear in children's eyes, medical experts busy at work, volunteers my daughter's age, and world leaders coming together on health issues.

What I have seen in the past 11 years tells me that even without cure for AIDS and easy treatment for MDR-TB, we can save lives and bring viral load to zero if we take the right action.

As I said in 2015 at the UN，a caring heart is our best weapon against AIDS. Fighting disease is an ongoing process, and it must be a joint effort. I'm grateful to WHO and UNAIDS for letting me be part of the great work you do and to my country's government for supporting my work as Goodwill Ambassador.

China has come a long way. It met the MDG for TB control five years ahead of schedule. It offers free HIV testing, free counseling and free treatment to cut mother-

常清楚如果我们不采取行动或行动不够及时,会导致什么样的后果。

自 2006 年以来,我走访了上述疾病的高发地区、偏远农村、医院、患者住所、社区中心、大中小学和研究机构,加深了对我们所面临的挑战的了解,并呼吁各方采取行动。我看到了孩子们眼中的痛苦和恐惧,目睹了医学专家忙碌工作的场景,见过许多和我女儿同龄的志愿者,也见证了各国领导人齐聚一堂探讨世界卫生问题的时刻。

过去十一年的所见所闻让我清楚地知道,尽管还未找到治愈艾滋病的办法,尽管治疗耐多药结核病的难度很大,但只要我们采取正确的措施,就能挽救生命,并将病毒载量降为零。

正如 2015 年我在联合国有关会议上所说,爱心是对抗艾滋病最好的武器。抗击疾病是一场持久战。这需要全世界的共同努力。非常感谢世卫组织和规划署,使我有机会参与你们所从事的伟大事业,也感谢我国政府支持我履行亲善大使的职责。

中国在抗击结核病与艾滋病方面已经取得了显著的成绩。中国提前五年实现了消除结核病的千年目标。中国政府向艾滋病患者提供免

to-child transmission. And it gives free education to AIDS orphans. As a result, fewer and fewer people die from the two diseases or suffer discrimination. China appreciates the help from WHO and UNAIDS and will remain your strong partner.

Through this job, I have witnessed how much the world can do together to make a difference. In December 2015, we invited 30 African AIDS orphans to a summer camp in Beijing. Seven months later, in July 2016, 30 African children and 30 Chinese children got together, and spent a wonderful week together. I watched them sing and dance, and made Chinese paper art with them. When I stood next to them and saw their smiling faces, I kept telling myself, whether these boys and girls can live a happy and healthy life will decide what our planet will look like. Knowing that these children will not be left behind gives us hope for an AIDS- and TB-free generation.

This is my 12th year advocating against TB and HIV/AIDS. It's a job that requires hard work, patience and devotion. I know my responsibility has increased, but so has my commitment and confidence. More and more people will join us in this important endeavor. It is not just a battle about the well-being of those affected. It is a battle

费的病毒检测、咨询服务以及母婴阻断药物,并免收艾滋孤儿的学费。如今,越来越少的人死于上述疾病或遭受社会歧视。中国赞赏世卫组织和规划署所给予的帮助,中国将永远是你们强有力的合作伙伴。

在担任亲善大使期间,我看到,只要大家携手合作,就能为这个世界带来积极的改变。2015 年 12 月,中方邀请 30 名非洲艾滋孤儿来华参加在北京举办的夏令营活动。七个月后,2016 年 7 月,30 名非洲儿童和 30 名中国儿童欢聚一堂,共同度过了一周的美好时光。我看着他们载歌载舞,并和他们一起体验了中国的剪纸艺术。站在他们身边,看着他们微笑的脸庞,我不禁对自己说:这些孩子能否拥有健康幸福的生活将决定我们这个星球未来的面貌。只要他们不被遗忘,我们就有希望实现"零艾滋、零结核"的目标。

今年是我宣传结核病和艾滋病防治的第十二个年头了。这项工作需要不懈的努力、极大的耐心和无私的奉献。我知道我的责任更重了,但我的决心和信心也更大了。我相信会有越来越多的人投身于这项崇高的事业。我们的努力不仅仅是为了帮助那些感染了疾病的人

about the future of humanity. We must succeed, and we will succeed.

This is what I would like to share with you today. Thank you.

们，更是为了确保人类能拥有更加美好的未来。我们必须成功，我们也一定能成功。

这就是我今天希望与各位分享的一些感想。谢谢大家。

Lecture 11　The Spellbinding Art of Human Anatomy

人体解剖——引人入胜的艺术

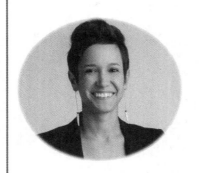

　　凡妮莎·鲁伊斯(Vanessa Ruiz)是一位医学插图家、用户界面设计者,也是解剖学的狂热爱好者。被人体解剖的动人之处所吸引,她于 2007 年建立了"Street Anatomy"(街头解剖)的博客,通过博文和艺术展览来告诉大众解剖是如何通过艺术、设计和流行文化的方式而被视觉化的。这在当时是一个创举。目前,医学插图已经打破了医学领域的范畴,正被艺术家和设计师广泛应用在自己的作品当中,以增加作品的人性要素。凡妮莎致力于向大众推介这些艺术家和他们将艺术与解剖相联系的创作方式。

1   As a lover of human anatomy, I'm so excited that we're finally putting our bodies at the center of focus. Through practices such as preventive medicine, patient *empowerment*① and self-monitoring—down to now obsessing over every single step we take in a day. All of this works promote a healthy connection between ourselves and our bodies.

2   Despite all this focus on the healthy self, general public knowledge of the anatomical self is lacking. Many people don't know the location of their vital organs, or even how they function. And that's because human anatomy is a difficult and *time-intensive*② subject to learn.

3   How many of you here made it through anatomy? Wow, good—most of you are in medicine. I, like you, spent countless hours memorizing hundreds of structures. Something no student of anatomy could do without the help of visuals. Because at the end of the day, whether you remember every little structure or not, these medical illustrations are what makes studying anatomy so intriguing. In looking at them, we're actually viewing a *manual*③ of our very selves.

1   作为一名人体解剖学的爱好者，很高兴看到大家终于开始将人体作为关注的焦点。通过不断的实践，诸如预防医学、患者授权和自我监督，直到日常生活的每一个细节，所有这一切都促进了我们自己和身体之间的健康关联。

2   然而大家关注的重点在健康本身，大众对解剖学仍然缺少一般的了解。很多人不知道自己的重要器官位于哪里，甚至不知道这些器官的功能是什么。这是因为人体解剖学是一门很难的学科，需要集中时间来学习。

3   在座有多少人是学过解剖的？哇，很棒，你们大多数都是医学生。和你们一样，我也花费了数不清的时间来记忆成百上千种结构。但是如果没有视觉辅助手段，没有任何一个学习解剖的学生能够完成这项任务。因为最后，无论你是否记住了每一个小结构，这些医学插图才是使得学习解剖如此迷人的原因。看着这些插图实际上就是看着我们自己

---

① empowerment *n.* 授权
② time-intensive *adj.* 费时的
③ manual *n.* 手册

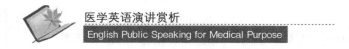

的身体手册。

4   But what happens when we're done studying? These beautiful illustrations are then shut back into the pages of a medical textbook，or an app，referenced only when needed. And for the public, medical illustrations may only be encountered passively on the walls of a doctor's office.

4   但是当我们学完这门课之后会怎样呢？这些美丽的插图只会被收入医学教科书或者应用程序当中，只有当需要时才会被查找出来。对于大众来说，可能只会在医生办公室的墙上瞥见这些医学插图。

5   From the beginnings of modern medicine，medical illustration，and therefore anatomy，have existed primarily within the realm of medical education. Yet there's something fascinating happening right now. Artists are breaking anatomy out of the *confines*① of the medical world and are *thrusting*② it into the public space. For the past nine years, I have been cataloguing and sharing this rise in anatomical art with the public—all from my perspective as a medical illustrator.

5   自现代医学诞生以来，医学插图，乃至解剖，主要存在于医学教育领域。但是一些有趣的事情正在发生。艺术家们将解剖带出了医学界，引入了公共领域。在过去的九年中，我一直在为解剖艺术编目分类并以一名医学插图家的角度将这种艺术的兴起分享给大众。

6   But before I get into showing you how artists are *reclaiming*③ anatomy today, it's important to understand how art influenced anatomy in the past.

6   但是在我向你们展示当代艺术家是怎样让解剖再生之前，有必要请大家先去理解在过去艺术是怎样影响解剖的。

---

①   confine *n.* 范围；界限
②   thrust *v.* 猛推；冲
③   reclaim *v.* 利用；改造

7   Now，anatomy is by its very nature a visual science，and the first anatomists to understand this lived during the **Renaissance**①. They relied on artists to help advertise their discoveries to their peers in the public. And this drive to not only teach but also to entertain resulted in some of the strangest anatomical illustrations.

8   Anatomy was caught in a struggle between science，art and culture that lasted for over 500 years. Artists **rendered**② dissected **cadavers**③ as alive，posed in these humorous anatomical **stripteases**④. Imagine seeing that in your textbooks today. They also showed them as very much dead—unwillingly stripped of their skin. **Disembodied**⑤ limbs were often posed in literal still lives. And some illustrations even included pop culture references. This is Clara，a famous rhinoceros that was traveling Europe in the mid-1700s，at a time when seeing a rhino was an exciting **rarity**⑥. Including her in this illustration was akin to celebrity sponsorship today.

7   解剖从本质上来说是一种视觉科学。文艺复兴时期的解剖学家们首先意识到这点。他们依赖艺术家的帮助去向自己的同行宣传自己的发现。教学和娱乐两大目标并存导致了一些奇怪的医学插图的诞生。

8   解剖陷入了一场科学、艺术和文化的战争，长达 500 多年。艺术家们将尸体绘制为鲜活的、摆出搞笑的脱衣舞姿势的解剖图。想象一下在现在的教科书里看到这些会怎样。他们也会让尸体呈现出死亡的样子——不情不愿地被剥掉了皮肤。失去躯干的四肢也经常被摆出活着的姿势。一些插图甚至会包括一些流行文化的内容。这是克拉拉，一头 18 世纪中期在欧洲巡回展演的犀牛。当时犀牛是让人激动的稀罕物。将犀牛画入插图就像今天请了一位名人来友情客串一样。

---

①   Renaissance *n.* 文艺复兴
②   render *v.* 提供
③   cadaver *n.* 尸体
④   striptease *n.* 脱衣舞（娘）
⑤   disembodied *adj.* 脱离肉体的
⑥   rarity *n.* 稀罕物

9　The introduction of color then brought a whole new depth and clarity to anatomy that made it stunning.

9　随后,色彩的引入为解剖带来了全新的深度和清晰度,使得它更加惊艳。

10　By the early 20th century, the perfect balance of science and art had finally been struck with the emergence of medical illustrators. They created a universal representation of anatomy—something that was neither alive nor dead, that was free from those influences of artistic culture. And this focus on no-frills accuracy was precisely for the benefit of medical education. And this is what we get to study from today.

10　在 20 世纪早期,伴随着医学插图家的出现,科学和艺术实现了完美的平衡。他们创造了解剖的通用表现模式——既不是生也不是死,且脱离了艺术文化的影响。它聚焦于毫无修饰的准确性上,使医学教育从中受益。而这也是我们现在要学习的地方。

11　But why is it that medical illustration—both past and present—captures our imaginations? Now, we are *innately*① tuned into the beauty of the human body. And medical illustration is still art. Nothing can *elicit*② an emotional response—from joy to complete disgust—more than the human body. And today, artists armed with that emotion, are grasping anatomy from the medical world, and are *reinvigorating*③ it through art in the most imaginative ways.

11　但是为什么不管是过去还是现在,医学插图都能激发我们的想象力呢? 我们天生就会被人体之美所吸引。医学插图仍然是艺术。没有什么能比人体更容易引起人们的情感反应——从欣喜到完全的厌恶。现在,被这些情感武装的艺术家们将解剖从医学领域带出,然后用最富有想象力的方式通过艺术使解剖复兴。

12　A perfect example of this is Spanish

12　西班牙当代艺术家费尔南

---

①　innately *adv.* 天生地
②　elicit *v.* 诱出;诱发
③　reinvigorate *v.* 使复兴;重振

contemporary artist Fernando Vicente. He takes 19th century anatomical illustrations of the male body and envelops them in a female *sensuality*①. The women in his paintings *taunt*② us to view beyond their surface anatomy, thereby introducing a strong *femininity*③ that was previously lacking in the history of anatomical representation.

13 Artistry can also be seen in the repair and recovery of the human body. This is an X-ray of a woman who *fractured*④ and *dislocated*⑤ her ankle in a roller-skating accident. As a tribute to her trauma, she commissioned Montreal-based architect Federico Carbajal to construct a wire sculpture of her damaged lower leg. Now, notice those bright red screws *magnified*⑥ in the sculpture. These are the actual surgical screws used in reconstructing her ankle. It's medical hardware that's been repurposed as art.

14 People often ask me how I choose the art that I showcase online or feature in gallery shows. And for me it's a balance between the

多·文森特就是一个完美的例子。他将 19 世纪医学插图中的男性身体用女性的感性重新诠释。他作品中的女性以一种嘲讽的方式，刺激我们透过解剖的表面看本质，从而创作出之前解剖史上所缺失的坚强的女性形象。

13　艺术也可以表现在对人体的修复上。这是一位女性的 X 射线图，她的脚踝在溜冰事故中脱臼骨折。为了给自己的创伤留个纪念，她委托蒙特利尔建筑师费德里科·卡瓦哈尔为她受伤的小腿做一个钢丝雕塑。注意一下雕塑中那些明亮的红色螺丝。这些就是在修复她的脚踝时所实际使用的螺丝。这是将医疗器械改用到艺术上的举措。

14　人们经常问我，如何选择艺术作品用于网上或画廊展示？对于我来说，重要的一点是要实现

① sensuality *n.* 感官；肉感
② taunt *v.* 嘲弄；讽刺
③ femininity *n.* 女性；妇女特质
④ fracture *v.* 骨折；断裂
⑤ dislocate *v.* 脱臼
⑥ magnify *v.* 放大；增强

technique and a concept that pushes the boundaries of anatomy as a way to know *thyself*①, which is why the work of Michael Reedy struck me. His serious figure drawings are often *layered*② in elements of humor. For instance, take a look at her face. Notice those red marks. Michael *manifests*③ the consuming insecurity of a skin condition as these *maniacal*④ cartoon monsters annoying and out of control on the background. On the mirrored figure, he renders the full anatomy and covers it in glitter, making it look like candy. By doing this, Michael *downplays*⑤ the common perception of anatomy so closely tied to just disease and death.

15 Now, this next concept might not make much sense, but human anatomy is no longer limited to humans. When you were a child, did you ever wish that your toys could come to life? Well, Jason Freeny makes those dreams come true with his magical toy dissections. One might think that this would bring a *morbid*⑥ edge to one's innocent childhood characters, but Jason says of his dissections, "One thing I've never seen in a child's reaction to my work

技术和概念之间的平衡,要让解剖成为大家了解自己的方式。这就是迈克尔·里迪打动我的原因。他的严肃的人物画经常含有幽默的元素。比如,看她的脸。注意那些红色的痕迹。迈克尔表现出强烈的糟糕的皮肤状况,就如同背景中那些讨厌的、失控的、癫狂的卡通怪兽。在镜像的身影上,他呈现了完整的解剖结构,并用光芒覆盖,使其看上去像糖果。通过这种方式,迈克尔淡化了解剖仅仅同疾病和死亡紧密相连的普遍观念。

15 下一个理念可能没什么意义,但是人类解剖并不再局限于人类。当你是个孩子的时候,你有没有希望过你的玩具能拥有生命? 那么,杰森·弗里尼的神器——解剖玩具,可以让你梦想成真。也许有人认为这会给天真无邪的童年带来病态的影响。但是当杰森提到他的解剖时,他说:"我从来没有在孩子对我作品的

---

① thyself *pron.* 你自己(第二人称反身代词,yourself 的古体)
② layer *v.* 分层堆放
③ manifest *v.* 表现;显现
④ maniacal *adj.* 狂野的;粗暴的
⑤ downplay *v.* 对……轻描淡写;弱化
⑥ morbid *adj.* 病态的

is fear." It's always wonder, amazement and wanting to explore. Fear of anatomy and guts is a learned reaction.

反应中看到恐惧。"孩子们展示的都是好奇、惊异和探索的欲望。对解剖和内脏器官的恐惧是后天习得的。

16　This anatomization also extends to politically and socially charged objects. In Noah Scalin's "Anatomy of War," we see a gun dissected to reveal human organs. But if you look closely, you'll notice that it lacks a brain. And if you keep looking, you might also notice that Noah has so thoughtfully placed the rectum at *the business end*① of that gun barrel.

16　解剖也会延伸到政治和社会的相关话题。在诺亚·斯卡林的作品《解剖战争》中，我们看到一把枪被打开，里面展示出人体的器官。但是如果你仔细观察，你会发现这把枪里没有大脑。如果继续观察的话，你也许还会注意到诺亚很有深意地把直肠放到了枪口。

17　Now, this next artist I've been following for many years, watching him excite the public about anatomy. Danny Quirk is a young artist who paints his subjects in the process of self-dissection. He bends the rules of medical illustration by inserting a very dramatic light and shadow. And this creates a 3 - D illusion that lends itself very well to painting directly on the human skin. Danny makes it look as if a person's skin has actually been removed. And this effect—also cool and *tattoo*②-like—easily transitions into a medical illustration. Now Danny is currently traveling the world,

17　接下来这位艺术家我关注了很多年，看着他激起了大众对解剖的热情。丹尼·夸克是一位年轻的艺术家，他擅长用自我解剖的手法作画。他打破了医学插图的常规，插入极具戏剧效果的光影，带来了三维效果，而这有助于直接在人体皮肤作画。丹尼的画作看起来好像真的去除掉了皮肤。这种效果很酷，看上去像文身，很容易转化成医学插图。目前丹尼正在环游世界，通过他的身体绘画将解剖传播给大众。所

---

① the business end（工具或武器）行使主要功能的一端

② tattoo *n.* 文身

teaching anatomy to the public via his body paintings, which is why it was so shocking to find out that he was rejected from medical illustration programs. But he's doing just fine.

18　Then there are artists who are extracting anatomy from both the medical world and the art world and are placing it directly on the streets. London-based SHOK-1 paints giant X-rays of pop culture icons. His X-rays show how culture can come to have an anatomy of its own, and conversely how culture can become part of the anatomy of a person. You come to admire his work because reproducing X-rays by hand, let alone with spray paint, is extremely difficult. But then again this is a street artist, who also happens to hold a degree in applied chemistry.

19　Nychos, an Austrian street artist, takes the term "exploded view" to a whole new level, *splattering*① human and animal dissections on walls all over the world. Influenced by comics and heavy metal, Nychos inserts a very youthful and *enticing*② energy into anatomy that I just love.

以当他被医学插图项目拒绝时，人们都感到非常震惊。但他照样享受现状。

18　还有一些艺术家们将医学领域和艺术领域中的解剖提取出来，然后直接将他们展示在街道上。伦敦的艺术家SHOCK－1绘制了关于流行文化的巨型X射线图。他的X射线图展示出文化如何拥有自己的解剖结构，而反过来文化又如何成为个人解剖的一部分。你不得不钦佩他的作品，因为用手工绘制X射线非常的困难，更不用说还要用喷漆的方式。不过碰巧的是他是一位拥有应用化学学位的街头艺术家。

19　奥地利街头艺术家尼克斯将"爆炸视图"发展到一个全新的水平。他将人和动物的解剖图涂鸦到世界各地的墙上。尼克斯受到漫画和重金属的影响，将青春和诱人的能量注入解剖当中，这是我所深深喜爱的。

---

① splatter *v.* 泼洒
② enticing *adj.* 诱人的；有吸引力的

[20] Street artists believe that art belongs to the public. And this street anatomy is so *captivating*① because it is the furthest remove from the medical world. It forces you to look at it, and confront your own perceptions about anatomy, whether you find it beautiful, *gross*②, morbid or awe-inspiring, like I do. That it elicits these responses at all is due to our intimate and often changing relationship with it.

[21] All of the artists that I showed you here today referenced medical illustrations for their art. But for them, anatomy isn't just something to memorize, but a base from which to understand the human body on a meaningful level; to *depict*③ it in ways that we can relate, whether it be through cartoons, body painting or street art.

[22] Anatomical art has the power to reach far beyond the pages of a medical textbook, to *ignite*④ an excitement in the public, and reinvigorate an enthusiasm in the medical

20　街头艺术家们认为艺术是属于大众的。街头解剖图是如此的诱人，因为这是解剖离开医学界最远的移植。你不得不去看，去审视自己对解剖学的看法，不管你认为它是美丽的、粗俗的、病态的或是像我一样觉得它是值得敬畏的。它之所以能激发这些情感，是因为我们同它之间的亲密的、经常发生变化的关系。

21　今天我介绍的所有的艺术家们，都在他们的艺术作品当中参考了医学插图的元素。但是对于他们来说，解剖并不仅仅是要去记忆的东西，而是一个基础。在这个基础上，人们在一个有意义的层面去理解人体，用一个可以关联我们的方式去描绘人体——不管是通过漫画、人体绘画还是街头艺术的方式。

22　解剖艺术的力量远远超出医学教科书，可以去点燃大众的激情和医学界的热情，最终将最深层的自我和人体联系起来。

---

①　captivating *adj.* 迷人的；有魅力的
②　gross *adj.* 粗俗的
③　depict *v.* 描述；描绘
④　ignite *v.* 点燃

world，ultimately connecting our *innermost*[①]   谢谢。
selves with our bodies through art. Thank you.

演讲赏析

这是一篇基于实物的说解性演讲（informative speech about objects）。演讲者从几个世纪前人体解剖艺术的发展谈起，介绍了一些将解剖和艺术融为一体的艺术家及其代表作品，旨在描述医学插图和当代艺术相辅相成的关系。因为面向普通的听众，话题又与相对枯燥和难懂的解剖学概念相关，演讲者没有过分注重对技术细节的解释，演讲内容也不涉及专业技术词汇，而是通过大量真实、生动的图片再现了人体解剖艺术这种视觉科学的生命力。这正是一篇说解性演讲的成功所在。

说解性演讲一般采用时间顺序法（chronological order）、空间顺序法（spatial order）和话题顺序法（topical order）来组织要点（main point）。本文的一大特色就是采用了两种要点组织方法。

在演讲的7—10段中，演讲者主要采用了时间顺序法来介绍不同历史阶段艺术对解剖学造成的影响。从文艺复兴时期到20世纪早期，医学插图的娱乐性和流行性的特点逐渐被严肃性和准确性所取代。

在演讲的12—20段中，演讲者的主要目的是介绍一些有特色的艺术家和他们的代表作品。因此，她采用了话题顺序法来组织要点。每一段主要介绍一位艺术家，每位艺术家就是演讲的一个要点。这样的内容安排结构清晰、层次分明、简单易懂。

除了要点组织法以外，本篇演讲的另一大特色是成功地使用了连接语（connectives）。在第6段，演讲者说："*But before I get into showing you how artists are reclaiming anatomy today，it's important to understand how art influenced anatomy in the past.*"这是一个典型的内部预展句（internal previews），可以让听众了解接下去要谈的内容。而第11段就是一个完整的过渡段（transition），自然而然地将话题从历史转到现在。

---

①   innermost *adj.* 最里面的；内心深处的

此外，演讲者使用了 PPT 作为视觉辅助手段（visual aids）。PPT 上并没有复杂的文字段落，而是一直呈现生动真实的图片。在这些图片的辅助下，听众可以更好地了解解剖艺术的发展，也会被人体解剖之美所深深吸引。

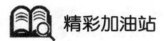 精彩加油站

On the Virtual Dissection Table
谈谈虚拟解剖台

精彩视频

You know, cadaver dissection is the traditional way of learning human anatomy. For students, it's quite an experience, but for a school, it could be very difficult or expensive to maintain. So we learned the majority of anatomic classes taught, they do not have a cadaver dissection lab. Maybe those reasons, or depending on where you are, cadavers may not be easily available.

So to address this, we developed with a Dr. Brown in Stanford: virtual dissection table. So we call this Anatomage Table. So with this Anatomage Table, students can experience the dissection without a human cadaver. And the table form is important, and since it's touch-interactive, just like the way they do dissections in the lab, or furthermore just the way a surgeon operates

大家知道，尸体解剖是学习人体解剖学的传统做法。对于学生来说，这是个非常好的体验机会，但是对于学校来说，遗体的供应很有难度，也很贵。所以据我们了解，大多数的解剖学课都没有尸体解剖的实践操作。可能是因为上述原因，或者因为地域原因，尸体解剖是不容易实现的。

为了解决这个问题，我们和斯坦福大学的布朗博士合作，开发了这个虚拟解剖台。我们把它叫做解剖影像台。用这个解剖台，学生们不需要真正的尸体就可以体验解剖。这个台面的设计很重要，它用的是触控技术，就跟在实验室里上解剖课一样，也可以像外科大夫给病人做手术一样，你可以和这个台

on a patient you can literally interact with your table. Our digital body is one-to-one life size, so this is exactly the way students will see the real anatomy.

I'm going to do some demonstrations. As you can see, I use my finger to interact with my digital body. I'm going to do some cuts. I can cut any way I want to, so I cut right here. Then it's going to show inside. And I can change my cut to see different parts. Maybe I can cut there, see the brain, and I can change my cut. You can see some internal organs. So we call this the slicer mode. OK, I'm going to do another cut. Right there. This shows a lot of internal structures. So if I want to see the back side, I can flip and see from behind. Like this. So if these images are uncomfortable to you or disturbing to you, that means we did the right job. So our doctors said these are eye candies.

So instead of just butchering the body, I'd like to do more clinically meaningful dissections. What I'm going to do is I'm going to peel off all the skin, muscles and bones, just to see a few internal organs. Right here. Let's say I'm going to cut the liver right here. OK. Let's say I'm interested in looking at the heart. I'm going to do some surgery here. I'm going to cut some veins, arteries. Oops! ... You don't want to hear "oops" in real surgery. （Laughter） But

子互动。这种数字化人体和真人一样大小，这使学生能够体验到真实的解剖情境。

我现在给大家做个示范。你们看，我可以用手指和这个数字人体互动。我现在要切了。我想怎么切都行，比如切这里。然后我们就看见内部了。想看其他部位，就切其他地方。我可以切这里来看大脑结构；也可以切那里去看腹内器官。这个功能叫切片模式。现在我在这里切一刀，就能看见内部的结构。如果我想看背部，我可以把身体翻过来，从背后看，就像这样。如果这些图像让你觉得不舒服或者恐惧了，那说明我们的工作成功了。我们的医生朋友就觉得这些图像挺赏心悦目的。

现在我不再随意地切来切去，我要展示一些有临床意义的解剖。我要剥去所有皮肤、肌肉和骨骼来观察一些内部器官。就是这里，我在肝脏的部位切下去。好了。如果我想了解心脏，我可以在这里做手术。我需要切割一些静脉和动脉。糟糕！在真正的手术中你可不想听到"糟糕"二字（笑声）。但幸运的是，这里我们可以撤销操作（笑声）。好了。

fortunately，our digital man has "undo." (Laughter) Okay.

All right then. Let me zoom in. I'm going to make a cut right there. And then you can see the inside of the heart. You can see the atrium and the ventricles, how blood flows to our arteries and veins. Just like this, students can isolate anybody and dissect any way you want to. It doesn't have to be always dissection. Since it's digital, we can do reverse dissection. So let me show you, I'm going to start with the skeletal structure, and I can add a few internal organs. Yep. Maybe I can add quickly this way. And I can build muscles gradually, just like that. We can see tendons and muscles. Wish I could build my muscle this fast. （Laughter） And this is another way to learn anatomy.

Another thing I can show you is, more often than not，doctors get to meet patients in X-ray form. So，Anatomage Table shows exactly how the anatomy will appear in X-ray. You can also interact with your X-ray, and also if you want，you can compare with how anatomy would appear in X-ray, too. So when you are done，just bring back the body and then it's ready for another session. It looks like our table also can transform gender，too. It's a female now.

So this is Anatomage Table. Thank you.

现在没问题了。让我放大来看,我就在这里切下去。然后你能看到心脏内部,看到心房和心室,看到血液是怎么流到动脉和静脉的。就像这样,学生们可以分离任何部位,用任何方法来解剖。它也不仅仅是为了解剖。因为这是数字的,我们可以做逆向解剖。我给你们展示一下。我们从骨架开始,加上几个内脏器官,就这样。我还能这样快速添加。再加上肌肉,一块一块加,就像这样。我们能看到肌腱和肌肉。真希望我自己的肌肉能长这么快(笑声)。这是另一种学习解剖的方式。

还有一个功能要展示一下。通常情况下,医生只能看见病人的 X 光片。而这个解剖台能展示人体在 X 光下看起来是什么样的。你还能和 X 光互动。如果你愿意,还能比较在 X 光下不同形式的解剖图。当你学习完了,把数字人体初始化,就可以用于下一节解剖课了。而且我们的解剖台还可以改变数字尸体的性别。现在变成女性了。

这就是我们的解剖影像台。谢谢大家。

Lecture 12   The Troubling Reason Why Vaccines Are Made Too Late
为什么疫苗姗姗来迟？

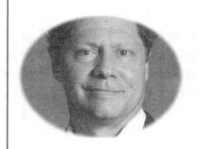

　　赛斯·伯克利（Seth Berkley）是一位著名的流行病学家，同时也是全球免疫疫苗联盟（The Global Alliance for Vaccines and Immunization，又称 GAVI）的 CEO。该组织是一个公私合作的全球卫生合作组织，成立于 1999 年，工作宗旨是与政府和非政府组织合作促进全球健康和免疫事业的发展。在 GAVI 的努力下，现在全球已有超过五亿的孩子接受了疫苗接种预防，而赛斯·伯克利希望 GAVI 可以在后面五年里再帮助三亿孩子获得疫苗接种，并使各国免疫项目获得更稳定持久的发展。在 2011 年加入 GAVI 之前，他还一直是 HIV 疫苗研制的倡导者，创立了国际艾滋病疫苗行动组织并担任其 CEO。赛斯·伯克利曾被《新闻周刊》列为封面人物，并在 2009 年入选《时代周刊》全球最具影响力 100 人。

1　The child symptom begins with mild fever, headache, muscle pains, followed by *vomiting*① and *diarrhea*②, then bleeding from the mouth, nose and *gums*③. Death follows in the form of organ failure from low blood pressure. Sounds familiar? If you're thinking this is Ebola, actually, in this case, it's not. It's an extreme form of *dengue fever*④, a mosquito-born disease which also does not have an effective *therapy*⑤ or a vaccine, and kills 22,000 people each year. That is actually twice the number of people that have been killed by Ebola in the nearly four decades that we've known about it. As for *measles*⑥, so much in the news recently, the death toll is actually tenfold higher. Yet for the last year, it has been Ebola that has stolen all of the headlines and the fear. Clearly, there is something deeply rooted about it, something which scares us and fascinates us more than other diseases. But what is it, exactly?

1　患儿的初始症状是低烧、头痛和肌肉疼痛。之后出现了呕吐和腹泻，后来口、鼻和牙龈开始出血。最终由于低血压引起了器官衰竭，导致死亡。是不是听起来很熟悉？也许你认为这是埃博拉病毒，可事实上，这起病例并不是。本例是登革热的极端形式，是一种通过蚊子传播的疾病，目前它也没有有效的治疗方法或者疫苗。每年有两万两千人死于这种登革热，而事实上，这个数字是我们知道埃博拉病毒以来的近四十年里埃博拉致死人数的两倍。而最近频现报端的麻疹造成的死亡病例实际上比埃博拉造成的死亡要多十倍。然而在过去一年来，却是埃博拉抢占了报纸头条，并引起了大面积恐慌。显然，埃博拉病毒的背后必然有些东西造成了我们的恐惧，并且让它比其他疾病更能吸引人们的关注。但这究竟是什么呢？

---

① vomit *v.* 呕吐
② diarrhea *n.* 腹泻
③ gum *n.* 牙龈
④ dengue fever *n.* 登革热
⑤ therapy *n.* 治疗方法
⑥ measles *n.* 麻疹

2　Well, it's hard to *acquire*① Ebola, but if you do, the risk of a horrible death is high. Why? Because right now, we don't have any effective therapy or vaccine available. And so, that's the clue. We may have it someday. We *rightfully*② fear Ebola because it doesn't kill as many people as other diseases. In fact, it's much less *transmissible*③ than viruses such as flu or measles. We fear Ebola because of the fact that it kills us and we can't treat it. We fear the certain *inevitability*④ that comes with Ebola. Ebola has this inevitability that seems to *defy*⑤ modern medical science.

2　其实,感染埃博拉并不是很容易,但你一旦被感染了,却极有可能以比较可怕的方式死去。为什么? 因为到目前为止,我们没有任何有效的治疗方法或者疫苗可以用。而这,正是原因所在,当然也许有一天我们会研制出来。所以我们害怕埃博拉是合情合理的,虽然它并没有其他疾病造成的死亡人数多,事实上,它比像流感、麻疹之类的疾病传染性低多了。我们害怕埃博拉主要是因为它可以杀死我们,而我们却无能为力。我们害怕的是感染埃博拉病毒会让死亡变得不可避免,而现代医学也束手无策。

3　But wait a second, why is that? We've known about Ebola since 1976. We've known what it's capable of. We've had *ample*⑥ opportunity to study it in the 24 *outbreaks*⑦ that have occurred. And in fact, we've actually had vaccine *candidates*⑧ available now for more than a decade. Why is it that those

3　但是,等一下,为什么会这样呢? 我们从 1976 年起就知道埃博拉病毒了,我们知道它有多厉害,我们也有足够的机会去研究这种病毒,因为已经有过 24 次疫情的爆发。而且事实上,我们手头上已经有了候选疫苗,并且在

---

① acquire *v.* 获得
② rightfully *adv.* 合情合理地
③ transmissible *adj.* 传染性的,可传染的
④ inevitability *n.* 不可避免性
⑤ defy *vt.* 藐视,违抗,使……不可能
⑥ ample *adj.* 足够的,充裕的
⑦ outbreak *n.* 爆发
⑧ candidate *n.* 候选者

vaccines are just going into *clinical trials*① now? This goes to the fundamental problem we have with vaccine development for *infectious*② diseases. It goes something like this: the people most at risk for these diseases are also the ones least able to pay for vaccines. This leaves little in the way of market *incentives*③ for manufacturers to develop vaccines, unless there are large numbers of people who are at risk in wealthy countries. It's simply too commercially risky. As for Ebola, there is absolutely no market at all, so the only reason we have two vaccines in late-stage clinical trials now, is actually because of a somewhat misguided fear. Ebola was relatively ignored until September 11 and the *anthrax*④ attacks, when all of a sudden, people perceived Ebola as, potentially, a bioterrorism weapon.

4   Why is it that Ebola vaccine wasn't fully developed at this point? Well, partially, because it was really difficult, or thought to be difficult, to weaponize the virus, but mainly because of the financially risk in developing it.

十多年以前就被研制出来了。那么为什么这些疫苗直到现在才进入临床试验? 这就涉及传染病疫苗研发中的一个根本问题。大致情况是这样的:患上该疾病风险最高的人群却也是最没有能力为其疫苗买单的人群。这就导致几乎没有市场动力来推动生产商研制疫苗,除非在富有国家有大量的人群面临感染风险。简单来说,它的商业风险太高了。而对于埃博拉病毒,根本毫无市场可言。所以现在我们能有两个疫苗进入到临床试验的最后阶段,唯一的原因其实是民众被误导的恐慌。在 911 事件和炭疽袭击之后,人们忽然意识到埃博拉是一种潜在的、具有生物恐怖袭击性的武器。而在此之前,相对于其他疾病,埃博拉并没有引起足够重视。

4   那么为什么埃博拉疫苗直到这个时候还没有被完全研制出来? 部分原因是因为这种病毒很难,或者说人们认为它很难被用做武器。但最主要的原因还是研

---

① clinical trial 临床试验
② infectious *adj.* 传染性的
③ incentive *n.* 刺激,奖励,激励
④ anthrax *n.* 炭疽病

And this is really the point. The sad reality is, we develop vaccine not based upon the risk the **pathogen**① poses to people, but on how economically risky to develop these vaccines. Vaccine development is expensive and complicated. It can cost hundreds of millions of dollars to take even a well-known **antigen**② and turn it into a **viable**③ vaccine.

制中的经济风险。这才是问题的关键所在。现实的可悲之处在于,我们研制一种疫苗首要考虑的并不是这种病原体对人类造成的威胁有多大,而是研制这种疫苗的经济风险有多大。疫苗研制既昂贵又复杂。选出一种抗原,甚至是已经熟知的抗原,将其转化为可用的疫苗,需要花费数亿美元。

5 Fortunately for diseases like Ebola, there are things we can do to remove some of the barriers. The first is to recognize when there's a complete market failure. In that case, if we want vaccines, we have to provide incentives or some type of **subsidy**④. We also need to do a better job at being able to figure out which are the diseases that most threaten us. By creating capabilities within countries, we then create the ability for those countries to create **epidemiological**⑤ and laboratory networks which are capable of collecting and **categorizing**⑥ these pathogens. The data from that then can be used to understand the

5 幸运的是,对于像埃博拉这样的疾病,我们还是可以做一些事情来打破这些壁垒的。首先需要认识到,市场的调控作用有时会失效。在这种情况下,如果我们还希望得到疫苗,就必须提供奖励措施,或进行某种形式的补贴。其次,我们也需要更好地弄清楚对我们威胁最大的疾病有哪些。通过在各国内建立研发团队,我们就可以让这些国家有能力建立流行病学和实验室网络,有了这些,我们就可以采集病原体,并进行分类。由此获得的数

---

① pathogen *n.* 病原体,致病菌
② antigen *n.* 抗原(能激发人体产生抗体)
③ viable *adj.* 切实可行的,可生存的
④ subsidy *n.* 补贴,补助金,津贴
⑤ epidemiological *adj.* 流行病学的
⑥ categorize *vt.* 把……分类

*geographic*① and *genetic*② diversity, which then can be used to help us understand how these are being changed *immunologically*③, and what type of reactions they promote.

据可以用来了解它们的地理分布和遗传多样性，帮助我们了解免疫学上的变化如何产生以及促进了哪种类型的反应。

6　So these are the things that can be done, but to do this, if we want to deal with a complete market failure, we have to change the way we view and prevent infectious diseases. We have to stop waiting until we see evidence of a disease becoming a global threat before we consider it as one. So, for Ebola, the *paranoid*④ fear of an infectious disease, followed by a few cases transported to wealthy countries, led the global community to come together, and with the work of dedicated vaccine companies, we now have these: two Ebola vaccines in *efficacy*⑤ trials in the Ebola countries, and a pipeline of vaccines that are following behind.

6　所以说，这些事情是可以做的。但是要做到这些，如果我们希望在市场无力的情况下解决问题的话，就必须改变我们看待和预防传染性疾病的方式。我们不能再等到某种疾病发展成为全球性的威胁之后，才开始正视这种疾病。因此，对于埃博拉病毒，正是由于有了对传染性疾病的极度恐慌以及几例传染者进入富国的病例，才使得全球各国携起手来。再加上疫苗公司的尽心工作，我们最终有了今天的结果——两种已经在发病国家进行疗效实验的埃博拉疫苗，而此后还会有更多的疫苗不断地被生产出来。

7　Every year, we spend billions of dollars, keeping a fleet of nuclear submarines permanently patrolling the oceans to protect us from a threat that almost certainly will never

7　每一年，我们都会花费数十亿美元以维持一支核潜艇舰队在海洋中巡逻，而这支舰队所防范的威胁，几乎可以肯定是不会出

---

① geographic *adj.* 地理学的
② genetic *adj.* 遗传学的
③ immunologically *adv.* 免疫地
④ paranoid *adj.* 多疑的，恐惧的，偏执狂的
⑤ efficacy *n.* 效力

happen. And yet, we spent virtually nothing to prevent something as *tangible*① and evolutionarily certain as epidemic infectious diseases. And make no mistake about it—it's not a question of "if", but "when." These bugs are going to continue to evolve and they are going to threaten the world. And vaccines are our best defense. So if we want to be able to prevent epidemics like Ebola, we need to take on the risk of investing in vaccine development and in *stockpile*② creation. And we need to view this, then, as the ultimate deterrent—something we make sure is available, but at the same time, praying we never have to use it. Thank you.

现的。但是，对于预防流行性传染病这样切实存在并不断进化的威胁，我们却不太舍得花钱。可别搞错了，它的发生并不是一个"如果"的问题，而是"什么时候"的问题。这些病毒还会不断进化，他们还将威胁整个世界，而疫苗正是我们最好的防御措施。所以如果我们想要预防类似于埃博拉这样的疫情，我们必须要承担起研制疫苗和建立储备的风险。我们应当把这看作最终的防线——我们要确保这条防线是有效的，但同时，我们也祈祷，永远不要用上它们。谢谢！

 演讲赏析

　　这是一篇有关政策的说服性演讲(persuasive speech on questions of policy)。演讲者以问题—成因—出路法(problem-cause-solution)的顺序展开论证，一步步地把听众引向自己的中心思想(central idea)：疫苗的研制往往不是由疾病的危害性决定的，而是由市场的利润推动的，我们必须要改变这一现状。

　　演讲的开头部分，演讲者用一段对疾病症状的描写使听众联想起最近颇受关注的埃博拉疫情。但他紧接着告诉大家一个令人吃惊的事实：本例并非大家熟知的埃博拉，而是登革热。选取这样一个震撼听众(startle the audience)的方法来作

---

　　① tangible *adj.* 有形的，实际的，可触摸的
　　② stockpile *n.* 囤聚的物资

为开篇,演讲者有效地激起了听众的好奇心(arouse the curiosity of the audience)。之后他又对听众提出了一个问题(question the audience):为什么埃博拉病毒比起其他致死疾病更容易引起人们的关注和恐慌?

通过回答这个问题,演讲者给出了自己的第一个论点(main point):*We fear Ebola because of the fact that it kills us and we can't treat it*. 紧接着,演讲者提出了第二个设问:为什么至今没有对抗埃博拉的疫苗问世? 通过回答这个问题,演讲者给出了自己的第二个论点(main point)——*We develop vaccine not based upon the risk the pathogen poses to people*,*but on how economically risky to develop these vaccines*。在这个因果推理论证(causal reasoning)的过程中,演讲者既采用了多次设问的方式来激发听众的思考,也通过各种数据(statistics),如第一段中各种疾病的死亡人数,以及事例(examples),如第三段的911、炭疽病毒等等,来支持自己的论证。当然,演讲者最终的目的并不仅仅是让听众被动地接受他的这个观点,他更希望自己的演讲可以带来一些实质性的改变,所以在之后一段,演讲者提出了几点改变现状的方法(solution)。

演讲的最后一段里,演讲者用类比推理的方法(analogical reasoning)进一步强化了自己的观点:我们在几乎用不上的核潜艇舰队上花费巨大,那么在传染病预防这样的问题上没有理由不增加投入。通过这样一层层的分析推理,演讲者已经在疫苗研制的迫切性以及增加投入的必要性这个问题上成功地说服了听众。

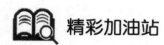 精彩加油站

Weekly Address：Taking Action Against the Zika Virus
美国总统奥巴马每周演讲——采取行动抗击塞卡病毒

精彩视频

Earlier this year, I got a letter from a South Carolina woman named Ashley, who

今年早些时候,我收到一封来自南卡罗来纳州女士的来信,她的

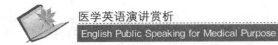
was expecting her third child. She was, in her words, "extremely concerned" about the Zika virus, and what it might mean for other pregnant women like her.

I understand that concern. As a father, Ashley's letter has stuck with me, and it's why we've been so focused on the threat of the Zika virus. So today, I just want to take a few minutes to let you know what we've been doing in response, and to talk about what more we can all do.

Since late last year, when the most recent outbreak of Zika started popping up in other countries, federal agencies like the Centers for Disease Control and Prevention have been preparing for it to arrive in the US. In February—more than six months ago—I asked Congress for the emergency resources that public health experts say we need to combat Zika. That includes things like mosquito control, tracking the spread of the virus, accelerating new diagnostic tests and vaccines, and monitoring women and babies with the virus.

Republicans in Congress did not share Ashley's "extreme concern," nor that of other Americans expecting children. They said no. Instead, we were forced to use resources we need to keep fighting Ebola, cancer, and other diseases. We took that step

名字叫艾希莉,马上就要迎接她的第三个孩子了。她的原话是,她"非常担心"塞卡病毒的传播,她不知道这个传染病对于她以及和她一样的怀孕女性意味着什么。

我能够理解这种担心。作为一个父亲,艾希莉的来信让我久久不能释怀,这也是我们一直关注塞卡病毒的原因。所以今天,我只想用几分钟的时间让大家了解一下我们政府已经采取的应对方案,以及我们所有人还可以采取的措施。

塞卡病毒的最近一次爆发是在去年晚些时候,当时其他国家接二连三受到波及。从那时起,疾控中心等联邦政府机构,就已经为其侵入做好了准备。二月份,即六个月以前,我和国会提出需要更多的应急资金,公共卫生专家认为这些是抗击塞卡病毒必需的。这些措施包括控制蚊虫数量,追踪病毒传播,更新诊断方法,加快疫苗研制,以及监察被感染孕妇。

可国会中的共和党人却没有艾希莉以及其他孕妇们那么忧心忡忡。他们拒绝采取行动,结果我们不得不把大量资金继续投入到埃博拉、癌症以及其他疾病的防治上去。我们迈出这一步,因为我们肩负着

because we have a responsibility to protect the American people. But that's not a sustainable solution. And Congress has been on a seven-week recess without doing anything to protect Americans from the Zika virus.

So my Administration has done what we can on our own. Our primary focus has been protecting pregnant women and families planning to have children. For months now, the CDC has been working closely with officials in Florida and other states. NIH and other agencies have moved aggressively to develop a vaccine. And we're working with the private sector to develop more options to test for and prevent infection. For weeks, a CDC emergency response team has been on the ground in South Florida, working alongside the excellent public health officials there—folks who have a strong track record of responding aggressively to the mosquitoes that carry viruses like Zika. They know what they're doing.

Still, there's a lot more everybody can and should do. And that begins with some basic facts.

Zika spreads mainly through the bite of a certain mosquito. Most infected people don't show any symptoms. But the disease can cause brain defects and other serious problems when pregnant women become

保护人民安全的重任。但现在的做法却并非长远之计。国会已经休会了七个礼拜，他们在抗击塞卡保护人民方面毫无作为。

因此我的政府已经采取了一切力所能及的措施。我们的工作重点是保护孕妇以及待孕家庭。疾控中心这几个月以来，一直在和佛罗里达州以及其他州的官员密切合作。国家卫生研究所等其他机构也在积极研制疫苗。我们目前正和一个私营机构合作，研发更多用于检测和防治的方法。几周以来，疾控中心的紧急应变工作队一直在南佛罗里达，和当地出色的公共卫生官员们一起奋战在一线——这些官员在对付病毒携带蚊虫方面战绩卓越。他们很清楚该怎么做。

此外，还有很多事是我们所有人都能够做的，也是应该做的。首先就是了解塞卡的基本情况。

塞卡病毒主要通过特定蚊虫的叮咬传播。大部分感染者不会出现任何症状。但孕妇被感染后，却会造成胎儿大脑损伤及其他严重问题。即使你不是孕妇，也不表示你

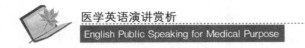

infected. Even if you're not pregnant, you can play a role in protecting future generations. Because Zika can be spread through unprotected sex, it's not just women who need to be careful—men do too. That includes using condoms properly.

If you live in or travel to an area where Zika has been found, protect yourself against the mosquitoes that carry this disease. Use insect repellant—and keep using it for a few weeks, even after you come home. Wear long sleeves and long pants to make bites less likely. Stay in places with air conditioning and window screens. If you can, get rid of standing water where mosquitoes breed. And to learn more about how to keep your family safe, just visit CDC.gov.

But every day that Republican leaders in Congress wait to do their job, every day our experts have to wait to get the resources they need—that has real-life consequences. Weaker mosquito-control efforts. Longer wait times to get accurate diagnostic results. Delayed vaccines. It puts more Americans at risk.

One Republican Senator has said that "There is no such thing as a Republican position on Zika or Democrat position on Zika because these mosquitoes bite everyone."

可以置身事外。因为塞卡可以通过无保护的性行为传播，这就意味着不仅仅女性需要小心行事，男性也不能例外。其中一个措施就是正确使用安全套。

如果你正居住在塞卡疫区，或打算去疫区旅行，请采取措施以防被携带病毒的蚊虫叮咬。你可以使用驱蚊产品，并在包括回家后的数周内持续使用。你也可以穿长袖长裤以降低叮咬概率。尽量待在有空调及纱窗的地方。有可能的话，清除可供蚊虫繁殖的积水。如果你还想了解更多信息保护家人，请登录CDC.gov官网查询。

每一天，国会里的共和党领导人都在拖延。每一天，我们的专家都在苦等所需资金——事关生死的资金。无效的蚊虫控制措施，漫长的确诊结果等待，迟到的疫苗，这一切的一切都在把美国人民置于危险之中。

一名共和党议员曾说："在塞卡病毒问题上，没有所谓的共和党政策或是民主党政策，因为蚊子咬人是不分党派的。"

I agree. We need more Republicans to act that way because this is more important than politics. It's about young mothers like Ashley. Today, her new baby Savannah is healthy and happy. That's priority number one. And that's why Republicans in Congress should treat Zika like the threat that it is and make this their first order of business when they come back to Washington after Labor Day. That means working in a bipartisan way to fully fund our Zika response. A fraction of the funding won't get the job done. You can't solve a fraction of a disease. Our experts know what they're doing. They just need the resources to do it.

So make your voices heard. And as long as I'm President, we'll keep doing everything we can to slow the spread of this virus, and put our children's futures first. Thanks everybody.

我很赞成。我们希望更多的共和党人可以这样表态,因为人民的健康比政治要重要得多。这样做正是为了像艾希莉一样的年轻母亲。现在她的孩子萨凡纳健康而又快乐,这才是重中之重。这也是为什么国会共和党人需要正视塞卡病毒的威胁,并在劳动节假期结束,回到华盛顿以后,立即着手处理此事。这意味着两党合作,共同资助塞卡病毒应对预案。只有部分资金是没有办法做到这些的,正如塞卡病毒也不可能只治疗一半。我们的专家知道该做什么,他们缺的只是资金。

所以请发出你们的呼声。只要我是总统,我们就会极尽所能延缓病毒传播,因为孩子的将来是一切之本。谢谢大家!

Lecture 13　Why Medicine Often Has Dangerous Side Effects for Women

药物对女性的副作用

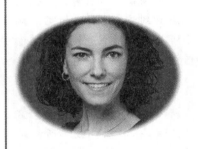

　　艾莉森·麦克格雷格（Alyson McGregor）博士是布朗大学沃伦·艾伯特医学院急诊医学系"急诊医学中的性和性别（SGEM）"（以前叫做"急诊护理中的女性健康"）课程的合作创始人和负责人。她的团队以急诊护理中的性与性别以及女性健康为研究内容，致力于该方面的教学与科研。McGregor 博士毕业于波士顿大学医学院并在布朗大学接受住院医师培训，随后在罗德岛医院急诊部任住院医师。她是急诊医学副教授，同时也是 SGEM 项目的共同负责人和"性和性别女性健康合作协会"这一全国性组织的合作创始人。

1　We all go to doctors. And we do so with trust and blind faith that the test they are ordering and the medications they're prescribing are based upon evidence—evidence that's designed to help us. However, the reality is that that hasn't always been the case for everyone. What if I told you that the medical science discovered over the past century has been based on only half the population?

1　我们生病都会去看医生，并且无条件地信任医生，相信他们做的检查和开的药都是有医学根据的，这样才对病人有益。然而事实上，这些并不适用于所有人。如果我告诉你，过去的一个世纪中，所有的医学发现只是基于一半的人群，你会怎么想呢？

2　I'm an emergency medicine doctor. I was trained to be prepared in a medical emergency. It's about saving lives. How cool is that? OK, there's a lot of runny noses and *stubbed*① toes, but no matter who walks through the door to the *ER*②, we order the same tests, we prescribe the same medication, without ever thinking about the sex or gender of our patients. Why would we? We were never taught that there were any differences between men and women.

2　我是急诊医生，学的就是如何处理各种急诊病情，挽救生命。听上去很酷，是不是？好吧，很多时候，我面对的是类似流鼻涕和踢伤脚趾的情况，但无论急诊病人是谁，我们都让他们做同样的检查，开同样的药，从不考虑病人的性别。为什么我们会这么做呢？因为我们从来没学过如何区别对待不同性别的病人。

3　A recent Government Accountability study revealed that 80 percent of the drugs withdrawn from the market are due to side effects on women. So let's think about that for a minute. Why are we discovering side effects on women only after a drug has been released to the

3　近期的一项政府问责研究表明，有80%的药物由于对女性会产生副作用而撤出市场。所以大家来想想，为什么在药物上市之后才发现它们对女性的副作用呢？你知道吗，药物上市要花费

① stub v. （脚趾）踢到
② ER　Emergency Room 急诊室

market? Do you know that it takes years for a drug to go from an idea to being tested on cells in a laboratory, to animal studies, to then clinical trials on humans, finally to go through a regulatory approval process, to be available for your doctor to prescribe to you? Not to mention the millions and billions of dollars of funding it takes to go through that process. So why are we discovering unacceptable side effects on half the population after that has gone through? What's happening?

4　Well, it turns out that those cells used in that laboratory, they're male cells, and the animals used in the animal studies were male animals, and the clinical trials have been performed almost exclusively on men.

5　How is it that the male model became our framework for medical research? Let's look at an example that has been popularized in the media, and it has to do with the sleep aid Ambien. Ambien was released on the market over 20 years ago, and since then, hundreds of millions of prescriptions have been written, primarily to women, because women suffer more sleep disorders than men. But just this past year, *the Food and Drug Administration* ① recommended cutting the dose in half for

多年时间，从一个简单的概念经过细胞实验、动物实验、人体临床试验、监管审批等一系列程序，才会出现在医生的处方上，给病人服用。更不用说在这一过程中高达上亿美元的投入。那为什么要到药物上市之后，我们才发现它们对一半的人群会产生副作用呢？这究竟是怎么一回事？

4　原因是细胞实验中用的都是雄性细胞，动物实验中用的是雄性动物，而临床实验的对象也几乎都是男性。

5　为什么雄性模型会成为医学研究的主体呢？让我们来看安眠药安必恩的广告。安必恩在二十多年前上市，卖出了成百上亿粒，服用者多为女性，因为患有睡眠障碍的女性比男性要多。但是就在去年，食品与药品监督局建议女性的服药量应减半，因为人们发现女性对该药物的代谢速度比男性慢，早晨起床后，药还会继续起作用，导致女性在驾车时昏昏

---

①　the Food and Drug Administration 美国食品药品管理局

women only，because they just realized that women *metabolize*① the drug at a slower rate than men，causing them to wake up in the morning with more of the active drug in their system. And then they're drowsy and they're getting behind the wheel of the car，and they're at risk for motor vehicle accidents. And I can't help but think，as an emergency physician，how many of my patients that I've cared for over the years were involved in a motor vehicle accident that possibly could have been prevented if this type of analysis was performed and acted upon 20 years ago when this drug was first released. How many other things need to be analyzed by gender? What else are we missing?

6　World War Ⅱ changed a lot of things，and one of them was this need to protect people from becoming victims of medical research without *informed consent*②. So some much-needed guidelines or rules were set into place，and part of that was this desire to protect women of *childbearing*③ age from entering into any medical research studies. There was fear：what if something happened to the fetus during the study? Who would be responsible? And so the scientists at this time actually thought this

欲睡，更容易发生车祸。作为急诊医生，我不禁会想，这些年来我处置的病人中，有多少出过车祸。如果在二十年前，药物上市前，人们发现了这一情况，这其中有多少车祸是可以避免的呢？而其他需要进行性别差异研究的药物又有多少？还有哪些是被我们遗漏的呢？

6　第二次世界大战带来了很多变化，对人的保护是其中之一，也就是说在把人体作为医学研究对象之前，要征得本人同意。为此，人们制定了一些法规，其中有一条是保护育龄女性，以防止其成为医学研究对象。因为科学家们害怕一旦实验对胎儿产生影响，要负担责任。他们也由此因祸得福，因为男性实验对象相对而言是同质的，他们的激素水平不会

---

① metabolize *v.* 新陈代谢
② informed consent 知情同意书
③ childbearing *n.* 生育

was *a blessing in disguise*①, because let's face it—men's bodies are pretty *homogeneous*②. They don't have the constantly *fluctuating*③ levels of *hormones*④ that could disrupt clean data they could get if they had only men. It was easier. It was cheaper. Not to mention, at this time, there was a general assumption that men and women were alike in every way, apart from their reproductive organs and sex hormones. So it was decided: medical research was performed on men, and the results were later applied to women.

7　What did this do to the notion of women's health? Women's health became *synonymous*⑤ with reproduction: breasts, *ovaries*⑥, *uterus*⑦, pregnancy. It's this term we now refer to as "bikini medicine." And this stayed this way until about the 1980s, when this concept was challenged by the medical community and by the public health policy makers when they realized that by excluding women from all medical research studies we actually did them a *disservice*⑧, in that apart

频繁波动，从而影响实验数据，所以采用男性实验对象更加简单，成本更低。此外，当时人们普遍认为除了生殖器官与性激素之外，男性与女性是相同的。所以事情就这么定了，采用男性作为医学实验对象，再把研究结果应用到女性身上。

7　这一决策对女性健康有什么影响呢？这就相当于把女性健康与乳房、卵巢、子宫、怀孕等联系在一起，等同于生殖健康，也就是我们现在所说的"比基尼医学"。这一概念的使用一直持续到20世纪80年代，医学界以及公共卫生政策制定者才对此提出质疑，他们意识到把女性排除在医学研究对象之外，会损害女性的利益，因为除了生育之外，女性病人的

---

① a blessing in disguise 因祸得福
② homogeneous *adj.* 同种类的
③ fluctuating *adj.* 波动的，起伏的
④ hormone *n.* 激素，荷尔蒙
⑤ synonymous *adj.* 等同于……的
⑥ ovary *n.* 卵巢
⑦ uterus *n.* 子宫
⑧ disservice *n.* 损害，伤害

from reproductive issues, virtually nothing was known about the unique needs of the female patient.

特殊需求根本无人了解。

8　Since that time, an overwhelming amount of evidence has come to light that shows us just how different men and women are in every way. You know, we have this saying in medicine: children are not just little adults. And we say that to remind ourselves that children actually have a different *physiology*① than normal adults. And it's because of this that the medical specialty of *pediatrics*② came to light. And we now conduct research on children in order to improve their lives. And I know the same thing can be said about women. Women are not just men with *boobs*③ and tubes. But they have their own *anatomy*④ and physiology that deserves to be studied with the same intensity.

8　从那时起,大量的证据开始涌现,证明男性与女性在各方面都完全不同。医学界有这样一个说法:儿童不是小号的成人。这样说是为了提醒我们,儿童的生理机能和正常的成人完全不同。为此,才把儿科设置成独立的医学专科。我们现在对儿童的专项研究是为了促进他们的健康。这同样适用于女性。女性并不是有乳房和卵巢子宫的男性。女性的生理构造同样也需要深入研究。

9　Let's take the *cardiovascular*⑤ system, for example. This area in medicine has done the most to try to figure out why it seems men and women have completely different heart attacks. Heart disease is the number one killer

9　以心血管系统为例,这一领域着眼于研究为何男性和女性的心脏病发作机制完全不同。心脏病是男性和女性共同的头号健康杀手,但和男性相比,更多的女性

---

① physiology *n.* 生理机能
② pediatrics *n.* 儿科
③ boob *n.* 乳房,胸部
④ anatomy *n.* 解剖
⑤ cardiovascular *adj.* 心血管的

for both men and women, but more women die within the first year of having a heart attack than men. Men will complain of crushing chest pain—an elephant is sitting on their chest. And we call this typical. Women have chest pain, too. But more women than men will complain of "just not feeling right," "can't seem to get enough air in," "just so tired lately." And for some reason we call this *atypical*①, even though, as I mentioned, women do make up half the population.

¹⁰ And so what is some of the evidence to help explain some of these differences? If we look at the anatomy, the blood vessels that surround the heart are smaller in women compared to men, and the way that those blood vessels develop disease is different in women compared to men. And the test that we use to determine if someone is at risk for a heart attack, well, they were initially designed and tested and perfected in men, and so aren't as good at determining that in women. And then if we think about the medications—common medications that we use, like aspirin. We give aspirin to healthy men to help prevent them from having a heart attack, but do you know that if you give aspirin to a healthy woman, it's actually harmful?

在首次发病后一年内死亡。男性患者多出现压迫性胸痛——好像有一头大象坐在胸口——我们把此称为典型症状。女性患者也会有胸痛，表现为"感觉不适""呼吸不畅""最近比较疲劳"等——但却被称为非典型症状。但正如我前面提到的，女性的人数要占到一半人口啊。

10　那么如何证明这些差异呢？从生理结构上看，女性心脏周围的血管比男性的要细，所以女性的血管相关疾病与男性不同。而我们筛查心脏病风险的检查专为男性设计，适用于男性，并不能有效地筛查女性罹患心脏病的风险。再看药物，常用药，以阿司匹林为例，健康男性可以服用阿司匹林来预防心脏病，但健康女性服用阿司匹林是否有害呢？

---

① atypical *adj.* 非典型的

¹¹ What this is doing is merely telling us that we are scratching the surface. Emergency medicine is a fast-paced business. In how many life-saving areas of medicine, like cancer and stroke, are there important differences between men and women that we could be utilizing? Or even, why is it that some people get those runny noses more than others, or why the pain medication that we give to those stubbed toes work in some and not in others?

¹² The Institute of Medicine has said every cell has a sex. What does this mean? Sex is DNA. Gender is how someone presents themselves in society. And these two may not always match up, as we can see with our *transgendered*① population. But it's important to realize that from the moment of conception, every cell in our bodies—skin, hair, heart and lungs—contains our own unique DNA, and that DNA contains the chromosomes that determine whether we become male or female, man or woman.

¹³ It used to be thought that those sex-determining chromosomes pictured here—XY if you're male, XX if you're female—merely determined whether you would be born with

11　可见我们的研究并不深入。急诊医学是快节奏的。在生死攸关的医学领域，如癌症和脑卒中，有多少性别差异是我们该引起重视的呢？或者为什么有些人得感冒的概率比别人高，为什么镇痛药对有些踢伤脚趾的人有效，而对另外一些人却无效呢？

12　医学研究所告诉我们每一个细胞都有性别之分。这意味着什么？性别就是 DNA。性别是每一个人在社会中表现出的样子。尽管对变性人来说，这二者可能并不一致。但我们必须认识到，从被孕育的那一刻开始，身体里的每一个细胞，包括皮肤、头发、心脏和肺，都含有独特的 DNA，而 DNA 所包含的染色体又决定了我们是雄性还是雌性，男人还是女人。

13　过去人们认为性染色体——男性是 XY，女性是 XX——决定了人身上长的是卵巢还是睾丸，而这些器官分泌的

---

① transgendered *adj.* 变性的

ovaries or *testes*①, and it was the sex hormones that those organs produced that were responsible for the differences we see in the opposite sex. But we now know that that theory was wrong—or it's at least a little incomplete. And thankfully, scientists like Dr. Page from the Whitehead Institute, who works on the Y chromosome，and Doctor Yang from UCLA，they have found evidence that tells us that those sex-determining chromosomes that are in every cell in our bodies continue to remain active for our entire lives and could be what's responsible for the differences we see in the dosing of drugs，or why there are differences between men and women in the *susceptibility*② and severity of diseases.

14   This new knowledge is the game-changer，and it's up to those scientists that continue to find that evidence，but it's up to the clinicians to start translating this data at the bedside，today. Right now. And to help do this, I'm a co-founder of a national organization called Sex and Gender Women's Health Collaborative，and we collect all of this data so that it's available for teaching and for patient care. And we're working to bring together the medical educators to the table. That's a big job. It's changing the way medical training has been

性激素造成了性别差异。但现在我们知道这一理论是错误的，至少是不太完整的。多亏了白头研究所的 Page 博士，他从事 Y 染色体研究，并和加州大学洛杉矶分校的杨博士合作，发现了性染色体会在人的一生中保持活跃，并由此产生在用药剂量、疾病的易感性以及严重性上的性别差异。

14   这一新发现改变了原有观念。科学家们的任务是继续研究找到证据。而临床医生则需要把新的数据转化运用到临床实践中，为此，我和同仁们成立了性和性别女性健康合作协会这一全国性组织，我们收集数据，将其运用到教学和病人护理中，并且正在和医学教育者合作。任务艰巨，但自从这一理论诞生以来，它正在改变着整个医学教育。

---

① testis *n.* 睾丸（复数为 testes）
② susceptibility *n.* 易感性

done since its *inception* ①.

¹⁵ But I believe in them. I know they're going to see the value of incorporating the gender lens into the current curriculum. It's about training the future health care providers correctly. And regionally, I'm a co-creator of a division within the Department of Emergency Medicine here at Brown University, called Sex and Gender in Emergency Medicine, and we conduct the research to determine the differences between men and women in emergent conditions, like heart disease and stroke and *sepsis* ② and substance abuse, but we also believe that education is *paramount* ③.

15　我坚信医学教育专家们会重视性别差异,并将其融入现有课程。这关系着未来医护人员的教育。我是布朗大学急诊医学一个部门的合作创始人,这个部门叫做急诊医学中的性和性别,主要研究性别差异在急诊中的体现,如心脏病、脑卒中、败血症、药物滥用等,我们认为开展相关学科教学的重要性不言而喻。

¹⁶ We've created a 360-degree model of education. We have programs for the doctors, for the nurses, for the students and for the patients. Because this cannot just be left up to the health care leaders. We all have a role in making a difference. But I must warn you: this is not easy. In fact, it's hard. It's essentially changing the way we think about medicine and health and research. It's changing our relationship to the health care system. But there's no going back. We now know just

16　我们构建了 360 度全方位的教学模型,为医生、护士、医学生以及病人分别开设了课程。因为这不仅仅是医疗保健领导者的任务,还需要我们每个人的努力。我必须提醒大家,任务并不轻松。事实上,任务非常艰巨,因为这会从根本上改变我们对医学、健康以及研究的思维方式,改变我们与医疗保健体系的关系。开弓没有回头箭,现在我们只知道我们

---

① inception *n.* 开端,开始
② sepsis *n.* 败血症
③ paramount *adj.* 首要的,至为重要的

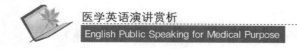

enough to know that we weren't doing it right.

过去做的并不对。

17 Martin Luther King, Jr. has said, "Change does not roll in on the wheels of inevitability, but comes through continuous struggle."

17　马丁·路德·金说过："改变不会自动到来，唯有不断抗争。"

18 And the first step towards change is awareness. This is not just about improving medical care for women. This is about personalized, individualized health care for everyone. This awareness has the power to transform medical care for men and women. And from now on, I want you to ask your doctors whether the treatments you are receiving are specific to your sex and gender. They may not know the answer—yet. But the conversation has begun, and together we can all learn. Remember, for me and my colleagues in this field, your sex and gender matter.

18　改变的首要步骤就是转变观念。这不仅仅意味着我们要改善女性医疗服务，而是要为每个人提供个性化的医疗服务，为男性和女性提供更好的健康服务。从现在开始，我希望你能问自己的医生，自己所接受的医疗服务是否已考虑到性别特征。医生可能也不知道答案。但交流既然已经开始，我们可以共同学习。请记住，对于我和我的同行而言，你的性别很重要。

19 Thank you.

19　谢谢！

 演讲赏析

　　这篇演讲涉及用药安全这一社会热点问题。一提到药物的副作用或用药安全，人们常会联想到用药剂量或用药不当产生的各种问题。很少有人会想到，男性和女性患者对相同的药物会有不同的反应。本篇演讲围绕这一话题展开，详细解释了性别差异对药物安全性产生的影响且着重分析其背后的原因,旨在唤起人们对这一问题的关注。

在这篇演讲中,演讲者采用设问(rhetorical questions)的方式,首先提出问题(problem):药物研发过程中的误区,接着揭示这一误区产生的原因(cause)、影响(effect)以及解决方法(solution)。各部分环环相扣,深入浅出又层层推进,让听众在听完演讲之后,对该问题有了全面而深入的了解。

首先,演讲者指出一个常常被人们忽视的事实:"过去的一个世纪中,所有的医学发现只是基于一半的人群"(*What if I told you that the medical science discovered over the past century has been based on only half the population*),她结合自己作为急诊医生的经历提出第一个问题:"为什么在诊疗中医生不会考虑病人的性别差异呢?"这就成功地引起了听众的兴趣(get attention and interest),想探究其背后的原因。接下来她告诉听众不仅在诊疗过程中,在药物的研发也存在同样的问题:为什么很多药物在上市之后才会因为发现对女性的副作用而撤回呢?围绕这一问题,她告诉听众,原来药品在研发过程中,用的都是雄性模型。那么为什么实验模型仅限于雄性呢?在分析了历史原因之后,她又指出:医学研究中仅用雄性模型作为医学试验和研究的对象,对女性健康会产生什么影响?紧随其后的一系列问题是:男性和女性的差异何在?这些差异由什么决定?意味着什么?在回答和分析这一系列问题的过程中,演讲者用事实(facts)和数据(statistics)佐证,让听众逐渐了解到医学研究中的性别差异,关注其带来的各种影响,并思考解决的对策。

演讲接近尾声,演讲者引用名人名言(quotation),用马丁·路德·金的话"改变不会自动到来,唯有不断抗争"(*Change does not roll in on the wheels of inevitability, but comes through continuous struggle*)来作为结尾部分的开始,以号召人们转变观念,再次唤起人们对医疗健康服务中性别差异的关注。

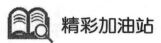

精彩加油站

Weekly Address：Trump's Attack on Obamacare
美国总统特朗普每周演讲：废除奥巴马医改方案

精彩视频

My fellow Americans,

Millions of families across our nation are suffering under the disaster known as Obamacare. Traveling throughout our country over the last two years, I have met so many of these wonderful Americans, and I have never forgotten their stories.

In Wisconsin, I recently met a proud Veteran and his wife—Michael and Tammy Kushman. When they were forced onto Obamacare and the exchange in 2015, they thought they would be able to keep their doctor—but they couldn't. They thought they would be able to keep their plan—but they weren't allowed. They were told their premiums would go down—but instead, they soared by 120 percent upward. It was one Obamacare lie after another. Today, the Kushmans spend ＄1,400 dollars a month on health insurance—nearly one-fourth of their entire net monthly income.

On the same visit, I met another family, Robert and Sarah Stoll. Robert is a volunteer

亲爱的美国同胞们：

数百万的美国家庭都在面临一场灾难，一场名为奥巴马医疗改革的灾难。在过去的两年里，我走遍全国各地，遇到了不少很棒的美国人民，他们背后的故事也给我留下了深刻的印象。

在威斯康星州，我遇到了一位自豪的老兵和他的妻子——迈克尔和塔米·库什曼。当他们被迫在2015年加入奥巴马医保的时候，他们本以为可以不换医生——但是他们失望了。他们本以为可以继续原来的医保计划——但是他们也被拒绝了。他们还听说保费会下调——可事实上他们的保费上涨了120%。奥巴马医改带来的谎言一个接着一个。现在，库什曼一家每个月在医保上的花费多达1 400美元——这几乎是他们每月家庭净收入的四分之一。

在这趟旅程中，我还遇到了另一个家庭，罗伯特和莎拉·斯托尔

captain for his local fire department. After their Obamacare premiums nearly doubled, they needed extra money and Sarah had no choice but to leave retirement to pay their bills. But this new income meant they were no longer eligible for the tax credit they had once received, and the federal government actually forced them to repay thousands and thousands of dollars.

These families and so many others are victims of a catastrophic law that is wreaking havoc on our healthcare system and our families.

Democrats in Congress created this calamity and now, if we don't act, millions more Americans will be hurt by Obamacare's deepening death spiral.

Americans were promised lower premiums, more choices, and better access. Instead, premiums have doubled nationwide, and insurers are still fleeing the market that Obamacare has nearly destroyed. Americans in nearly one-third of all counties have only one insurer to choose from on the exchanges—and many markets may soon have no insurers at all. It really is a disaster.

The American people are calling out for relief, and my administration is determined

一家。罗伯特是当地消防局的志愿者队长。他们的保费在奥巴马医保之后几乎翻倍了,为了支付这笔额外的开销,莎拉不得不放弃退休重新工作。这笔新的收入意味着他们没有资格再享受之前的税收减免,实际上联邦政府的做法使他们不得不重复支付数千美元。

这些家庭以及其他类似的家庭都是一部糟糕法律的受害者,它对我们的医疗体系以及无数家庭而言无异于一场灾难。

正是国会中的民主党人一手制造了这场灾难,而如果我们现在还不采取行动的话,奥巴马医改这场愈演愈烈的死亡旋涡还将波及数百万美国人民。

我们的人民在这场改革中得到的承诺是他们的保费会更低,选择会更多,就医也会更便捷。可实际上保费在全国范围内翻倍了,而因为医改的破坏,保险公司也在不断退出市场。全美几乎三分之一县的市场上,只有一家保险公司可选——有的甚至就要面临无公司可选的局面。这实在是一场巨大的灾难。

美国人民需要帮助,我的政府也决心伸出援手——我们现在正和

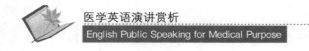

to provide it—and we are working with Congress to get a bill to my desk so we can rescue Americans from this catastrophe.

As families across the nation continue to suffer under this law, I only hope that Democrats in Congress will have the political courage to help fix what we know to be a catastrophic situation—a total disaster—that they have created, to be part of the solution, instead of obstructing—always obstructing—change, blocking reform, and doubling down on Obamacare's failure.

But no matter what, my Administration will never stop fighting for you—and for the healthcare system that you deserve. We'll get it done. Even if we don't have any help from the Democrats, we'll get it done.

Thank you, God bless you, and God bless America.

国会一起努力，以期通过一个法案，把美国人民从这场灾难中解救出来。

目前全美的无数家庭仍在因为奥巴马的法案备受煎熬，我只希望国会的民主党人能有足够的政治勇气来修正这糟糕的局面——一场由他们一手造成的灾难。而作为解决方案的一部分，也希望他们可以不要再阻挠改变，妨碍变革，在医改的失败上一错再错。当然，阻挠也是他们一贯的作风了。

但是不管怎样，我的政府绝不会停止为你们而努力，为你们应该享有的医疗体系而努力。我们会成功的。即使没有来自民主党人士的帮助，我们依然会成功。

谢谢你们！愿上帝保佑你们！愿上帝保佑美国！

Lecture 14　What Makes Life Worth Living in the Face of Death

当死亡降临

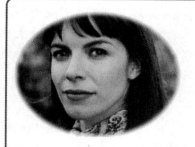

　　露西·卡拉尼什（Lucy Kalanithi）是斯坦福医院的一名内科医生。她的丈夫保罗曾是一名神经外科医生，从不吸烟的他在年仅 36 岁时即被确诊为四期肺癌，并于两年后去世。在治疗阶段，保罗提笔写下了他的回忆录《当呼吸化为空气》（*When Breath Becomes Air*）。凭借他斯坦福大学文学学士和硕士的语言功力，保罗用优美动人的语言记录了自己从医生向病人转变过程中的点点滴滴感悟。虽然这本书的结尾部分不得不由他的妻子也是校友兼同事——露西帮他完成，但依然位列美国畅销书排行榜第一。他的妻子露西在保罗生命的最后阶段一直陪伴左右，这段痛苦而特别的旅程让同为医生的她对生命有了不同的感悟，从此她便致力于提升病人的临终体验，帮助病人做出合理也合情的医疗选择。也许对于她而言，保罗的去世是结局，也是开始。

1　A few days after my husband Paul was diagnosed with stage Ⅳ lung cancer, we were lying in our bed at home, and Paul said, "It's going to be OK." And I remember answering back, "Yes." We just don't know what OK means yet.

2　Paul and I had met as first-year medical students at Yale. He was smart and kind and super funny. He used to keep a gorilla suit in the trunk of his car, and he'd say, "It's for emergencies only."

3　I fell in love with Paul as I watched the care he took with his patients. He stayed late talking with them, seeking to understand the experience of illness and not just its technicalities. He later told me he fell in love with me when he saw me cry over an *EKG*① of a heart that had ceased beating. We didn't know it yet, but even in the heady days of young love, we were learning how to approach suffering together.

4　We got married and became doctors. I was

1　就在我丈夫保罗被确诊为肺癌晚期的几天后，我们躺在家里的床上，保罗说："一切会变好的。"我记得我的回答是"是的"。我们当时并不知道变好意味着什么。

2　保罗和我是在耶鲁医学院一年级的时候认识的。他聪明、友善，而且超有幽默感。他曾经在他的汽车后备厢里放了一件大猩猩的服装，他的说法是："紧急情况时能用得上。"

3　当我目睹了他细心照顾病患的情景之后便爱上了他。他会和病患聊到很晚，试图去理解疾病给个人带来的感触，而不是技术层面的细节。他后来告诉我，当他看到我面对一张心电图，因为病人心脏停止跳动而变成一条直线，便忍不住哭泣的那一刻，就爱上了我。我们那时并不知道，即使年轻的我们正处于头脑发热的热恋期，却已经在学着如何一起面对痛苦了。

4　我们结婚了，毕业后都成为

---

①　EKG (electrocardiogram) *n.* 心电图

working as an *internist* ① and Paul was finishing his training as a neurosurgeon when he started to lose weight. He developed excruciating back pain and a cough that wouldn't go away. And when he was admitted to the hospital, a *CT scan* ② revealed tumors in Paul's lungs and in his bones. We had both cared for patients with devastating diagnoses; now it was our turn.

5   We lived with Paul's illness for 22 months. He wrote a memoir about facing *mortality* ③. I gave birth to our daughter Cady, and we loved her and each other. We learned directly how to struggle through really tough medical decisions. The day we took Paul into the hospital for the last time was the most difficult day of my life. When he turned to me at the end and said, "I'm ready," I knew that wasn't just a brave decision. It was the right one. Paul didn't want a *ventilator* ④ and *CPR* ⑤. In that moment, the most important thing to Paul was to hold our baby daughter. Nine hours later, Paul died.

了医生。我做了内科医生,而保罗正要结束他的神经外科训练课程,可他的体重也在此时开始下降。他的后背疼得厉害,而咳嗽也总是不见好。当他被收治住院时,CT 显示肿瘤已经到了肺和骨头里。我们都照顾过身患重病的病人,现在,轮到我们自己了。

5   我们和保罗的病魔斗争了22个月。在这期间,他写了一本回忆录,记录面临死亡的感受。我们的女儿卡迪出生了,我们很爱她,也很爱彼此。我们学会了如何在各种两难的医学方案中做出痛苦的选择。我最后一次把保罗送去医院的那天是我一生中最艰难的一天。他在最后一刻转向我,对我说:"我已经准备好了。"那一刻,我知道这不仅仅是一个勇敢的决定,也是正确的选择。保罗不想用呼吸机和心肺复苏。在那一刻,对保罗而言最重要的事是抱着我们襁褓中的女儿。九个小时之后,保罗走了。

---

① internist *n.* 内科医师
② CT scan 电脑断层扫描
③ mortality *n.* 必死性,必死的命运
④ ventilator *n.* 呼吸机
⑤ CPR (cardiopulmonary resuscitation) 心肺复苏术

6   I've always thought of myself as a caregiver—most physicians do—and taking care of Paul deepened what that meant. Watching him reshape his identity during his illness, learning to witness and accept his pain, talking together through his choices—those experiences taught me that *resilience*① does not mean bouncing back to where you were before, or pretending that the hard stuff isn't hard. It is so hard. It's painful, messy stuff. But it's the stuff. And I learned that when we approach it together, we get to decide what success looks like.

6   一直以来，我认为自己是懂看护的——大部分医生都是这么想的——而照顾保罗的经历却让我对这一角色有了更深刻的认识。目睹他在病程中转换自己的角色，学会认识并接受自己的痛苦，和他一起商量并做出决定，这些经历都让我意识到，坚强并不意味着回到之前的状态，或是装作所有困难都没什么大不了的。困难就是困难，它必然会带来痛苦和麻烦，你不用否认。我慢慢明白了，当我们一起面对困难时，我们必须重新理解成功的定义。

7   One of the first things Paul said to me after his diagnosis was, "I want you to get remarried." And I was like, whoa, I guess we get to say anything out loud.

7   保罗在确诊后对我说的第一句话就是"我希望有一天你能再找个人嫁了"。我当时就觉得，天哪，看来我们什么事都得挑明了说了。

8   It was so shocking and heartbreaking—and generous, and really comforting because it was so *starkly*② honest, and that honesty turned out to be exactly what we needed. Early in Paul's illness, we agreed we would just keep saying things out loud. Tasks like making a will, or completing our advance directives—

8   这种做法让人非常惊讶和难受——但却也显得大度和贴心，因为这才是彻底的坦诚，而这种坦诚正是我们所需要的。在保罗患病的早期，我们就说好，一切事情都要敞开了说。像是立遗嘱，或是预留医疗指示——那些我一

---

①   resilience *n.* 适应力，复原力
②   starkly *adv.* 严酷地，毫无掩饰地

tasks that I had always avoided—were not as *daunting*① as they once seemed. I realized that completing an advance directive is an act of love—like a wedding vow. A pact to take care of someone, *codifying*② the promise that till death do us part, I will be there. If needed, I will speak for you. I will honor your wishes. That paperwork became a tangible part of our love story.

9   As *physicians*③, Paul and I were in a good position to understand and even accept his diagnosis. We weren't angry about it, luckily, because we'd seen so many patients in devastating situations, and we knew that death is a part of life. But it's one thing to know that; it was a very different experience to actually live with the sadness and uncertainty of a serious illness. Huge *strides*④ are being made against lung cancer, but we knew that Paul likely had months to a few years left to live.

10   During that time, Paul wrote about his transition from doctor to patient. He talked about feeling like he was suddenly at a crossroads, and how he would have thought

直在逃避的事——其实并没有想象的那么可怕。我意识到预留医疗指示是一种爱的举动——就像婚礼上的誓言一样。我们承诺要照料对方，我们写下我们的誓言，直到生死相隔，永不言弃。我将会在需要时为你表达你的意愿，完成你的愿望。这一纸契约成为我们爱情故事的见证。

9   作为医生，保罗和我都能够很好地理解甚至去接受诊断结果。很幸运，我们没有愤怒，因为我们见过太多的危重病人，我们知道死亡也是生命的一部分。但知道是一回事，而真正身患重病、经历悲痛和各种不确定却是另一回事了。尽管对肺癌的治疗方法已经有很大的进步，但我们依然知道保罗能活着的日子只有几年，甚至几个月了。

10   在这个阶段，保罗把自己从医生到病人的转变记录了下来。他说道，感觉自己就像忽然被扔到了一个十字路口，本以为自己

---

① daunting *adj.* 令人生畏的
② codify *v.* 将……编成法典
③ physician *n.* 内科医生
④ stride *n.* 步幅，进步

he'd be able to see the path, that because he treated so many patients, maybe he could follow in their footsteps. But he was totally *disoriented*①. "Rather than a path," Paul wrote, "I saw instead only a harsh, vacant, gleaming white desert. As if a sandstorm had erased all familiarity. I had to face my mortality and try to understand what made my life worth living, and I needed my oncologist's help to do so."

11 The *clinicians*② taking care of Paul gave me an even deeper appreciation for my colleagues in health care. We have a tough job. We're responsible for helping patients have clarity around their *prognoses*③ and their treatment options, and that's never easy, but it's especially tough when you're dealing with potentially *terminal*④ illnesses like cancer. Some people don't want to know how long they have left, others do. Either way, we never have those answers. Sometimes we substitute hope by emphasizing the best-case scenario. In a survey of physicians, 55 percent said they painted a rosier picture than their honest opinion when describing a patient's prognosis.

可以看清眼前的道路,因为他也曾治疗过那么多的病人,也许跟着他们的脚步自己也可以看到未来的方向。可是他却彻底地迷失了。"根本不是一条路,"保罗写道,"我看到的只有一片荒芜、空虚、亮得晃眼的白色沙漠,就好像我所熟悉的一切都已经被一场沙尘暴扫荡干净。我不得不面对我即将死亡的现实,努力搞清自己生命的意义,这个过程,我都离不开我的肿瘤医生的帮助。"

11　保罗的临床医生对他的照料加深了我对医疗界同事的感激。我们的工作很难。我们有义务帮助患者清楚知道疾病的预后和他们可以有的医疗选择,这向来就不是简单的事,尤其是在处理癌症这样的不治之症的时候。有的人不想知道他们自己还有多少时日,有的人却正好相反。可不管是哪种,我们都不会知道答案。有时候我们会强调最好的可能性,让希望听上去更大一些。在一次面向医生的调查中,百分之五十五的医生说当他们跟病人描述预后的时候,会说得比他们

① disoriented *adj.* 分不清方向或目标的
② clinician *n.* 临床医生
③ prognosis *n.* 预后(复数为 prognoses)
④ terminal *adj.* 晚期的,终点的

It's an instinct born out of kindness. But researchers have found that when people better understand the possible outcomes of an illness, they have less anxiety, greater ability to plan and less trauma for their families.

的真实想法听上去更美好一些。这是一种善意的本能。但研究者却发现,当患者可以更清楚地了解到疾病的预期后果时,他们反而不再那么焦虑,他们可以更好地做规划,而对家庭来说也意味着更少的痛苦。

12   Families can struggle with those conversations, but for us, we also found that information immensely helpful with big decisions. Most notably, whether to have a baby. Months to a few years meant Paul was not likely to see her grow up. But he had a good chance of being there for her birth and for the beginning of her life. I remember asking Paul if he thought having to say goodbye to a child would make dying even more painful. And his answer astounded me. He said, "Wouldn't it be great if it did?" And we did it. Not in order to spite cancer, but because we were learning that living fully means accepting suffering.

12   一个家庭在讨论这类话题时,可能非常痛苦,但对我们而言,我们却发现真实信息在需要做出重大决策时也是非常重要的。其中最值得一提的就是,要不要生一个孩子。保罗的预期寿命只有几个月到几年,这意味着他不可能看到孩子长大。但是他也许有机会看到女儿的出生,并在她生命的开始阶段陪伴左右。我记得问过保罗,和孩子离别会不会让死亡变得更痛苦。他的回答令我很震惊。他说:"真这样不是很好吗?"于是我怀孕了。我们这么做并不是为了和癌症斗争,而是因为我们明白了接受痛苦也是完整生活的一部分。

13   Paul's oncologist tailored his chemo so he could continue working as a neurosurgeon, which initially we thought was totally impossible. When the cancer advanced and Paul shifted from surgery to writing, his

13   保罗的肿瘤医生适量减少了他的化疗剂量,这样他还可以

*palliative care*① doctor *prescribed*② a *stimulant*③ medication so he could be more focused. They asked Paul about his priorities and his worries. They asked him what trade-offs he was willing to make. Those conversations are the best way to ensure that your health care matches your values. Paul joked that it's not like that "birds and bees" talk you have with your parents, where you all get it over with as quickly as possible, and then pretend it never happened. You revisit the conversation as things change. You keep saying things out loud. I'm forever grateful because Paul's clinicians felt that their job wasn't to try to give us answers they didn't have, or only to try to fix things for us, but to counsel Paul through painful choices ... when his body was failing but his will to live wasn't.

继续他的神经外科的工作，而我们在一开始觉得这是完全不可能的。当他的癌症进一步加重时，就不能再继续外科工作了，于是保罗又开始了写作。他的姑息疗法医生给他开了兴奋类的药物，这样他可以更专注地写作。他们询问了保罗最在意的事和最担心的事。他们也问了他在一些需要取舍的问题上的意见。这些谈话可以更好地确保你的医疗方案符合你最根本的意愿。保罗开玩笑地说，这可不像是你和你父母之间关于性启蒙问题的谈话，那种谈话大家都是有多快能多快地赶紧结束，然后假装什么也没发生。这些谈话却不是这样。每当情况发生变化，你就得重温这些对话。你得一直把一切真实地、明白地说出来。我会永远感激保罗的临床医生，因为他们从不觉得他们的工作是给我们一个连他们自己都不知道的答案，或是仅仅试着为我们把一切恢复原状，而是在保罗面临痛苦的选择时给予咨询和建议……当他的身体日渐衰弱，而他精神却依然矍铄。

---

① palliative care 姑息治疗，临终关怀
② prescribe *v.* 开处方
③ stimulant *n.* 兴奋剂

14　Later, after Paul died, I received a dozen bouquets of flowers, but I sent just one—to Paul's oncologist, because she supported his goals and she helped him weigh his choices. She knew that living means more than just staying alive.

15　A few weeks ago, a patient came into my clinic. A woman dealing with a serious *chronic*① disease. And while we were talking about her life and her health care, she said, "I love my palliative care team. They taught me that it's OK to say 'no'." "Yeah," I thought, "of course it is." But many patients don't feel that. Compassion and Choices did a study where they asked people about their health care preferences. And a lot of people started their answers with the words "Well, if I had a choice …" If I had a choice. And when I read that "if," I understood better why one in four people receives excessive or unwanted medical treatment, or watches a family member receive excessive or unwanted medical treatment. It's not because doctors don't get it. We do. We understand the real psychological consequences on patients and their families. The thing is, we deal with them, too. Half of critical care nurses and a quarter of *ICU*② doctors have considered quitting their jobs because of distress

14　在保罗死后，我收到了很多束花，但我只送出去一束——给保罗的肿瘤医生的，因为她支持保罗实现了他的目标，并且帮助他权衡已有的选择。她知道生活不仅仅意味着活着。

15　几周前，一位病人来到我的诊所，一位患有严重慢性病的女士。当我们聊到她的生活和医疗时，她说："我爱我的姑息治疗小组的医生们，是他们让我知道我可以说'不'。"是啊，我想，我们当然可以说不，可很多患者却没有意识到这点。一个名为"Compassion and Choice"的组织曾做过一个研究，当人们被问及他们的医疗倾向时，很多人的回答都是以"嗯，如果我有选择的话……"开头的。如果我有选择。当我读到这个"如果"时，我才更加理解了为什么每四个人中就有一个人接受了过度医疗，或是目睹一个家庭成员接受这样的治疗。并不是因为医生不知道，我们都知道。我们了解这一做法会对患者和他的家人带来的实际心理影响。问题是，我们也有自己的困扰要处理。有半数的重症监

---

①　chronic *adj.* 慢性的，长期的
②　ICU (Intensive Care Unit) 重症加护病房

over feeling that for some of their patients, they've provided care that didn't fit with the person's values. But doctors can't make sure your wishes are respected until they know what they are.

护护士和四分之一的 ICU 医生考虑过换工作，因为他们也知道自己提供的护理有时候和患者的根本意愿是相悖的，这种感觉让他们非常痛苦。但是只有当医生知道你的意愿是什么，才有可能尊重它们。

16 Would you want to be on life support if it offered any chance of longer life? Are you most worried about the quality of that time, rather than quantity? Both of those choices are thoughtful and brave, but for all of us, it's our choice. That's true at the end of life and for medical care throughout our lives. If you're pregnant, do you want *genetic screening*①? Is a knee replacement right or not? Do you want to do *dialysis*② in a clinic or at home? The answer is: it depends. What medical care will help you live the way you want to? I hope you remember that question the next time you face a decision in your health care. Remember that you always have a choice, and it is OK to say no to a treatment that's not right for you.

16 你是否愿意通过生命维持装置延续你的生命？那时的你是更关注生命的质量，还是生命的长度？这两种选择在临终和日常医疗中都会遇到。但无论选择了哪一个，都是病患在深思熟虑后的勇敢决定。这是患者自己的选择。如果你怀孕了，你想做基因筛查吗？要不要更换膝关节？你希望在家还是在诊所做血液透析？这一切问题的答案是：看情况。哪种医疗方案能够帮助你按你想要的方式生活？我希望你在下一次面对你的医疗方案选择时，能够记得问自己这个问题。记住，你始终可以选择。而且当医疗方案不适合你时，你可以说"不"。

17 There's a poem by W. S. Merwin—it's just

17 默温曾写过一首诗——很

---

① genetic screening 基因筛检
② dialysis *n.* 血液透析

two sentences long—that captures how I feel now. "Your absence has gone through me like thread through a needle. Everything I do is stitched with its color." For me that poem evokes my love for Paul, and a new *fortitude*① that came from loving and losing him.

18 When Paul said, "It's going to be OK," that didn't mean that we could cure his illness. Instead, we learned to accept both joy and sadness at the same time; to uncover beauty and purpose both despite and because we are all born and we all die. And for all the sadness and sleepless nights, it turns out there is joy. I leave flowers on Paul's grave and watch our two-year-old run around on the grass. I build bonfires on the beach and watch the sunset with our friends. Exercise and mindfulness meditation have helped a lot. And someday, I hope I do get remarried.

19 Most importantly, I get to watch our daughter grow. I've thought a lot about what I'm going to say to her when she's older. "Cady, engaging in the full range of experience—living and dying, love and loss—is

短，只有两行——却正好描述了我现在的感受。"你的离去如一条丝线，穿过了我。那些思念，一针一针，缝缀着我的每一天。"对于我而言，这首诗唤起了我对保罗的爱，以及在经历了爱和失去后学会的坚毅。

18　当保罗说"一切都会好的"，这并不意味着他的癌症能够痊愈。然而在这一段经历中，我们学会了去接受快乐还有悲伤，学会了去发现生活中的美好和意义，因为我们虽来到这个世界，但都终将离开，这一切都无法回避。其实在那些悲伤的不眠之夜以外，也有着快乐的时光。我会在保罗的墓前摆上一束鲜花，看着我们两岁大的孩子在草地里奔跑玩耍。我会在海滩边点起篝火，和朋友一起看日落。健身和冥想是很有帮助的。我想某一天我也真的会再次走入婚姻的殿堂。

19　最重要的是，我能够看着女儿一天天长大。我一直在思考，当她再大一些的时候我该如何让她明白这个道理。"卡迪，去拥抱人生的一切吧——生与死，爱与

---

① fortitude *n.* 坚毅，勇气

what we get to do. Being human doesn't happen despite suffering. It happens within it. When we approach suffering together, when we choose not to hide from it, our lives don't diminish, they expand."

失去——这都是我们必须要经历的。我们身而为人，无法回避苦难。痛苦是人生的一部分。当我们能够一起面对它，当我们选择不再去回避，我们的生活并不会崩塌，而是会慢慢好起来的。"

20 I've learned that cancer isn't always a battle. Or if it is, maybe it's a fight for something different than we thought. Our job isn't to fight fate, but to help each other through. Not as soldiers but as shepherds. That's how we make it OK, even when it's not. By saying it out loud, by helping each other through ... and a gorilla suit never hurts, either.

20　经历过这些我才知道治疗癌症并不是一场战役。或者说如果是的话，可能也是一场跟我们的想象不同的战役。我们要做的不是跟命运抗争，而是相互扶持，渡过难关。我们不需要像战士一样作战，而是要像牧羊人一样去照料。即使疾病并不一定会"好起来"，但我们确实可以让生活"好起来"。开诚布公，相互扶持，这一段旅程终将过去……当然备上一套大猩猩戏服也没坏处。

21 Thank you.

21　谢谢大家。

演讲赏析

这是一篇说服性演讲(persuasive speech)。演讲者以平缓而优美的语调娓娓叙述了她在丈夫保罗患肺癌期间一段痛苦的心路历程。通过对这段经历的回忆和反思,她希望更多的听众可以接受一个观点,面对医疗选择,患者应当真实地了解预后并做出最符合自己期望的决定。

开篇部分,演讲者先以说故事(tell a story)的口吻叙述了自己和身患癌症的丈夫保罗之间的一段对话,这一做法立刻吸引了听众的注意力(get attention and interest),快速地把听众拉入了自己的演讲话题之中。随后对于自己和丈夫如何相遇相恋的回忆,既是一段背景介绍,也很自然地让听众了解了演讲者本人和丈夫的职业——医生,这一身份无疑为下面的说服部分增加了可信度(establish credibility)。

在后面的主体部分,演讲者先以病患家属的身份,叙述了绝症病人所承受的肉体和精神上的痛苦,又从医生的角度解释了处理这种情况的医疗惯例和医生面临的两难局面。在这个过程中,演讲者既用到了当事者证言(peer testimony),例如第 10 段中引用的保罗所说的话(*Rather than a path, I saw instead only a harsh, vacant, gleaming white desert. As if a sandstorm had erased all familiarity.*),也用到了一些单项数据(single statistics),例如 11 段中解释医疗现状时,提到 55%的医生都会美化疾病的预后问题。此外在演讲的后半部分,演讲者又用了一个延展例证(extended example),详细叙述了她本人所遇到的一名病患在接受了姑息治疗后发出的感叹和自己的领悟(第 15 段),从而最终引出了自己的论点:*Remember that you always have a choice, and it is OK to say no to a treatment that's not right for you*(第 16 段)。这种从例子到结论的推理方法就是说服性演讲中常用的归纳法(reasoning from specific instances)。

在演讲的结尾部分,演讲者先是引用(quotation)了默温的一首短诗表达自己的心境,然后又以首尾呼应(refer to the introduction)的方式重新回到演讲开头她和保罗的对话以及保罗在汽车后备厢里藏着大猩猩戏服这两件事上去。这种结尾方式既让人感到温暖,又深化了自己的论点。

演讲者的语言运用也很值得借鉴。不管是明喻(simile),例如第 20 段关于牧羊人(shepherds)的比喻,还是排比(parallelism),例如第 19 段对女儿说的一段话

(Cady, engaging in the full range of experience—living and dying, love and loss—is what we get to do. Being human doesn't happen despite suffering. It happens within it. When we approach suffering together, when we choose not to hide from it, our lives don't diminish, they expand.)，这些优美的语言都有效淡化了死亡这一残酷的主题，并深深打动了听众，利用情感诉求（appealing to emotions），增添了情绪感染力，进一步提升了整篇演讲的说服效果。

纵观整篇演讲，演讲者的说服部分自然、真诚而富有感染力。她所使用的技巧——建立信誉度（building credibility）、使用证据（using evidence）、运用推理方法（reasoning）和利用情感诉求（appealing to emotions）——正体现了亚里士多德提出的论辩三要素（ethos, logos, and pathos）在说服过程中的重要性。

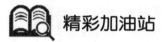 ## 精彩加油站

"Am I dying?" The Honest Answer
"我快死了吗?"一个诚实的回答

精彩视频

I've been a critical care EMT for the past seven years in Suffolk County, New York. I've been a first responder in a number of incidents ranging from car accidents to Hurricane Sandy.

If you are like most people, death might be one of your greatest fears. Some of us will see it coming. Some of us won't. There is a little-known documented medical term called impending doom. It's almost a symptom. As

过去七年，我在纽约州萨福克郡做一名医疗急救员。作为先遣急救员，我处理过一系列的事故现场，有车祸，也有飓风桑迪。

和大多数人一样，死亡可能是你最深切的恐惧。当死亡来临时，有人会意识到，有些人则不会。医学上有个很少为人知晓的术语叫做"濒死状态"。这种状态更像是一种

a medical provider, I'm trained to respond to this symptom like any other, so when a patient having a heart attack looks at me and says, "I'm going to die today," we are trained to reevaluate the patient's condition.

Throughout my career, I have responded to a number of incidents where the patient had minutes left to live and there was nothing I could do for them. With this, I was faced with a dilemma: Do I tell the dying that they are about to face death, or do I lie to them to comfort them? Early in my career, I faced this dilemma by simply lying. I was afraid. I was afraid if I told them the truth, that they would die in terror, in fear, just grasping for those last moments of life.

That all changed with one incident. Five years ago, I responded to a motorcycle accident. The rider had suffered critical, critical injuries. As I assessed him, I realized that there was nothing that could be done for him, and like so many other cases, he looked me in the eye and asked that question: "Am I going to die?" In that moment, I decided to do something different. I decided to tell him the truth. I decided to tell him that he was going to die and that there was nothing I could do for him. His reaction shocked me to this day. He simply laid back and had a look of acceptance on his face. He was not met

症状。作为医护人员，我接受了培训，学习如何像应对其他症状一样面对这种状态。当病人心脏病发作，看着我对我说："我今天要死了，"我们要知道如何重新评估病人的状况。

在我的职业生涯中，曾经多次遇到这样的情况：病人还剩下几分钟的生命，我已无力回天。所以面对这样的困境：我该不该告诉他，他快要死了呢？或者可以用谎言来安慰他？在刚从事这行的时候，我都用谎言来安慰病人。我很担心，担心如果告诉他们真相，他们会在恐惧中死去，在生命的最后时刻挣扎痛苦。

一次事故让我改变了做法。五年前，我去处理一场摩托车事故。车手伤得非常严重，做了检查后，我意识到自己救不了他，而他像很多病人一样，看着我的眼睛问我："我是不是快死了？"那一刻，我做出了与以往不同的决定。我决定告诉他真相。我决定告诉他他快要死了，而我帮不了他。直到今天，他的反应还是令我震惊。他平静地躺着，脸上是接受了现实的表情。他没有像我所想象中那样表现出恐惧和害怕。他就这样躺着，我从他的眼中看到的是平静和对现实的接受。从

with that terror or fear that I thought he would be. He simply laid there, and as I looked into his eyes, I saw inner peace and acceptance. From that moment forward, I decided it was not my place to comfort the dying with my lies. Having responded to many cases since then where patients were in their last moments and there was nothing I could do for them, in almost every case, they have all had the same reaction to the truth, of inner peace and acceptance. In fact, there are three patterns I have observed in all these cases.

The first pattern always kind of shocked me. Regardless of religious belief or cultural background, there's a need for forgiveness. Whether they call it sin or they simply say they have a regret, their guilt is universal. I had once cared for an elderly gentleman who was having a massive heart attack. As I prepared myself and my equipment for his imminent cardiac arrest, I began to tell the patient of his imminent demise. He already knew by my tone of voice and body language. As I placed the defibrillator pads on his chest, prepping for what was going to happen, he looked me in the eye and said, "I wish I had spent more time with my children and grandchildren instead of being selfish with my time." Faced with imminent death, all he wanted was forgiveness.

那一刻起,我决定不再用谎言来安慰将死的病人。从那天起,我发现在我无能为力,病人濒临死亡的情况下,几乎所有的病人对死亡做出了相同的反应——内心平静,安然接受。事实上,我发现他们的反应会有三种。

第一种反应总是会让我吃惊。无论病人宗教信仰或文化背景如何,他们总要祈求宽恕。他们或觉得自己有罪,或对某件事后悔,无一例外地都有着负疚感。一次,我抢救一位心脏病严重发作的老人,在我准备仪器,应对即将发生的心跳骤停的时候,我开始告诉他死亡将要来临。他其实已经从我的语气和动作里知道了什么。我把除颤器放在他胸口,为将要发生的事做准备,他看着我的眼睛,对我说:"我很自私,把很多时间都用在了独处上,要是能多陪陪儿孙们就好了。"面临死亡时,他所想得到的只是宽恕。

The second pattern I observe is the need for remembrance. Whether it was to be remembered in my thoughts or their loved ones', they needed to feel that they would be living on. There's a need for immortality within the hearts and thoughts of their loved ones, myself, my crew, or anyone around. Countless times, I have had a patient look me in the eyes and say, "Will you remember me?"

The final pattern I observe always touched me the deepest, to the soul. The dying need to know that their life had meaning. They need to know that they did not waste their life on meaningless tasks.

This came to me very, very early in my career. I had responded to a call. There was a female in her late 50s severely pinned within a vehicle. She had been t-boned at a high rate of speed, critical, critical condition. As the fire department worked to remove her from the car, I climbed in to begin to render care. As we talked, she had said to me, "There was so much more I wanted to do with my life." She had felt she had not left her mark on this Earth. As we talked further, it would turn out that she was a mother of two adopted children who were both on their way to medical school. Because of her, two children had a chance they never would have had otherwise and would go on to

第二种反应是需要被怀念。如果能被我或是被他们爱的人怀念，他们就会觉得自己的生命得到了延续。他们需要永远活在他们所爱的人、我、我的同事们或任何人的心中。无数次，病人看着我的眼睛，对我说："你会记得我吗？"

最后一种反应让我感触最深，直达我的灵魂深处。垂死的人渴望知道自己生命的意义。他们想知道自己没有在无意义的事情中虚度人生。

在我刚开始从业的时候，接到一次急救任务，有个年近六十的女士，由于从侧面而来的高速撞击，被卡在车里。消防员正忙着把她从车里救出来，我爬进车里开始急救。她对我说："我这一辈子还有很多想做的事情。"她觉得自己活着的时候没有在世上留下印记。在我们的谈话中，我慢慢知道她曾收养了两个孩子，而且都要去读医学院。因为她，两个孩子获得了本不可能得到的机会，以后会成为医生救死扶伤。把她从车里救出来花了45分钟，而她在被解救出来之前就停止了呼吸。

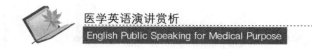
save lives in the medical field as medical doctors. It would end up taking 45 minutes to free her from the vehicle. However，she perished prior to freeing her.

I believed what you saw in the movies：when you're in those last moments that it's strictly terror，fear. I have come to realize，regardless of the circumstance，it's generally met with peace and acceptance，that it's the littlest things，the littlest moments，the littlest things you brought into the world that give you peace in those final moments.

Thank you.

我以前相信电影里所看到的场景：处在生命的最后时刻里，人会非常害怕、非常恐惧。而现在，我认识到，无论在什么情形下，人都能平静地接受死亡，而正是生命中那些最微不足道的事情和最微不足道的时刻，以及你为这个世界带来的最微不足道的变化，让你在生命的最后时光里得到平静。

谢谢！